COVID-19
Global Pandemic and Aspects of Human Security in South Asia
Implications and Way Forward

COVID-19
Global Pandemic and Aspects of Human Security in South Asia
Implications and Way Forward

Delwar Hossain

Md. Shariful Islam

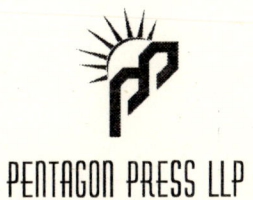

PENTAGON PRESS LLP

COVID-19 Global Pandemic and Aspects of Human Security in South Asia: Implications and Way Forward

By Delwar Hossain, Md. Shariful Islam

ISBN 978-93-90095-08-7

First Published in 2020

Copyright © RESERVED

All rights reserved. No part of this publication may be reproduced, stored in a retrieval system, or transmitted in any form or by any means, electronic, mechanical, photocopying, recording or otherwise, without the prior written permission of the Publisher.

Disclaimer: The views and opinions expressed in the book are the individual assertion of the Authors. The Publisher does not take any responsibility for the same in any manner whatsoever. The same shall solely be the responsibility of the Authors.

Published by
PENTAGON PRESS LLP
206, Peacock Lane, Shahpur Jat,
New Delhi-110049
Phones: 011-64706243, 26491568
Telefax: 011-26490600
email: rajan@pentagonpress.in
website: www.pentagonpress.in

Printed at Aegean Offset Printers, Greater Noida, U.P.

CONTENTS

	Preface	ix
1	**Introduction**	1
	Understanding COVID-19 Global Pandemic and Human Security	3
	Understanding Human Security	4
2	**Health Security in South Asia**	11
	Introduction	11
	Theorising Health Security	12
	State of Health Security in South Asia	14
	Privatisation of Healthcare and Growing Inequalities	*20*
	COVID-19 and Vulnerability of South Asian Health System	22
	Implications of COVID-19 in South Asian Health Security	23
	Affecting the General Patients	*24*
	Diverting Critical Resources to Fight COVID-19	*25*
	Mental Health Ramifications	*25*
	Disrupting Regular Immunisation Services	*27*
	Remittances and Health (In)security	*27*
	COVID-19, Violence and Conflicts	*28*
	Possible Policy Responses	30
	Individual as Referent Object of Security	*30*
	Investing more on Health	*30*
	Improving Disease Surveillance Systems in Humans and Animals	*30*
	Addressing Inequalities	*31*
	Role of Non-state Actors	*31*
	Focusing on Diplomacy	*31*
	Role of Individuals	*32*
	Role of Scholars and Scholarship	*32*
	Conclusion	32
3	**Food Security in South Asia**	39
	Introduction	39

	Understanding Food Security	40
	Dimensions of Food Security	*41*
	Food Security in South Asia: A Brief Account	42
	Implications of COVID-19 on Food Security	44
	COVID-19 and Food Security in South Asia	47
	Food Availability	*48*
	Accessibility of Food	*51*
	Nutrition Access and Food Utilisation	*54*
	What is to be Done	55
	Prioritising Agriculture	*55*
	Stabilising Food System and Keeping Trade Open	*56*
	Strengthening Economy	*57*
	Strengthening Social Safety Net Programmes	*57*
	Promoting Regional Cooperation	*57*
	Conclusion	58
4	**Economic Security in South Asia**	**63**
	Introduction	63
	Theorising Economic Security	66
	State of Economic Security in South Asia	69
	Threats to Economic Security in South Asia	*72*
	COVID-19 and South Asian Economy	76
	Implications for South Asian Economic Security	79
	Poverty	*80*
	Inequality	*80*
	Lives and Livelihoods	*81*
	Some Positive Trends	*83*
	Policy Responses	84
	Conclusion	86
5	**Environmental Security in South Asia**	**91**
	Introduction	91
	Conceptualising Environmental Security	94
	Key Environmental Challenges in South Asia	95
	Air Pollution	*96*
	Climate Change	*99*
	Marine Plastic Pollution	*100*
	Soil Degradation	*102*
	COVID-19 and Environment in South Asia	102
	Air Pollution	*103*
	Climate Change	*105*
	Implications for South Asian Environmental Security	108
	Policy Imperatives	111
	Focusing on Environmentally Sensitive Climate Policy	*111*
	Promoting Renewable Energy and other Low-carbon Sources	*111*
	Mainstreaming Air Pollution	*112*

	Reinforcing Regional Initiatives	113
	Ending North-South Divide in Global Environmental Politics and Reducing Emissions	114
	Conclusion	114
6	**COVID-19 and Regional Cooperation in South Asia: Challenges and Possibilities**	**121**
	Introduction	121
	An Overview of Growth of Cooperation in South Asia	124
	SAARC-Centrism	126
	Sub-regional/Inter-regional Cooperation	127
	Low Level of Economic Integration	128
	Politico-Strategic Cooperation	128
	Role of Civil Society	129
	Regionalism and Globalisation	130
	Relevance of Regional Response to COVID-19	131
	COVID-19 Focused Initiatives	133
	New Prospects and Old Challenges	136
	Conclusion	140
7	**COVID-19 and the Crisis of Global Health Governance: Implications for South Asia**	**145**
	Introduction	146
	Theorising Global Health Governance	147
	Narratives on Global Health Governance: A Brief Account	149
	COVID-19 Global Pandemic: A Crisis of Global Health Governance	154
	Failure of the Norm of Cooperation	155
	Crisis of Global Leadership	157
	Marginalisation of the World Health Organisation	159
	Marginalisation of Science from Policy Processes	160
	Implications for South Asia	161
	Looking Ahead	164
	Prioritising Health	165
	Promoting International Cooperation and Innovations	165
	Strengthening the Role of WHO	166
	Role of the Rising Powers	166
	Role of Epistemic Communities: Bring Science and Scientists Back in Policy Processes	167
	Rethinking Contemporary World Politics	167
	Conclusion	169
8	**Conclusion: Way Forward**	**174**
	Index	180

PREFACE

Since the end of the 1918-22 Spanish Flu global pandemic, the world has never witnessed such a large-scale and multidimensional human disaster. Data from various sources such as Johns Hopkins University Coronavirus Resource Centre and Worldometers.info show that the virus has affected 213 countries and territories in the world. More than ten million people have been infected by COVID-19 while about 500,000 people have died in this pandemic. South Asian countries have been suffering hugely from COVID-19. India, Pakistan and Bangladesh lead the curve of COVID-19 infected people in the region. Although preventive measures of South Asian countries have generally contained the spread and fatalities from COVID-19, it has had a profound impact on every sector of human activity ranging from the economic to education.

In particular, livelihoods and public health systems have been worst affected by COVID-19. The talk of a New Normal in the post-COVID-19 era gives some sense of understanding the impact of this crisis on South Asia. Hence, there is a need for a study of the implications of COVID-19 for human security in order to fathom the emerging theoretical and policy issues in the region. This book attempts to understand the impact of a critical and emerging issue called the COVID-19 global pandemic that South Asia has been facing today. It aims to provide critical analysis and insights on this contemporary challenge to policy makers, health professionals, academics, students, researchers, NGO workers working with health, human security and everyone interested in health and human security in South Asia. It covers major human security areas, i.e., health security, food security, economic security, and the environment issue. The role of regional cooperation and global health governance is also covered in the domain of COVID-19.

The idea of this book first originated in a conversation with my young colleague and a former student, Md. Shariful Islam, about the COVID-19 pandemic. We were discussing how fast it had transformed our world almost in the blink of an eye. Perhaps, no force on earth in the form of war or natural disaster could have such a colossal impact on human society in this short span of time. Initially, it came as a serious health issue at a personal level. People became worried about their individual life. The focus was to survive the attack of the novel coronavirus. Social distancing, physical distancing, wearing masks, collecting personal protective equipment (PPE), and many other different preventive measures have captured the imagination of the people. Disturbing reports such as children abandoning parents and vice versa due to COVID-19 started to appear in mainstream and social media. Rumours and a spree of hatred were gradually becoming headlines of newspapers in South Asia. This reflected how people thought about the problem so much at a personal scale. South Asian values based on family and collectivism have suffered.

Interestingly, in the initial weeks of the COVID-19 pandemic, South Asia witnessed a lesser number of infections, almost negligible in number. People also argued that the region would remain outside of the gravity of the COVID-19 pandemic attack. From climate to culture, every aspect of South Asian life was mentioned as a reason behind possible immunity of the region from the COVID-19 pandemic. However, everything was proved wrong. Gradually, the number of infected people has increased and spiked in the region. It has skyrocketed from a small figure like a few thousands to about a million in almost six weeks. It has soon become crystal clear that the challenge of COVID-19 is multifarious. It has impacted every sector and 'everyday life' of people. From psychological trauma to economic slowdown at national, regional and global levels, everything has been deeply affected by the COVID-19 pandemic. In this cataclysmic change in reality, the 'individual' comes first.

We had immediately thought about human security as a relevant perspective to focus on this work. Since it is an evolving context, we have selected major aspects of human security to understand the impact of the COVID-19 pandemic. Of course, South Asia immediately comes as a region to our mind. Since its decolonisation in the late 1940s, South Asia has witnessed wars, ethnic conflicts, communal riots, military coups, assassinations of national leaders, natural disasters such as floods, cyclones, droughts and earthquakes, nuclearisation, and terrorism. The COVID-19 pandemic has been added to the list of challenges that the region is facing in its cruellest and most destructive way, which was unimaginable even in mid-2019.

Our sincerest thanks are to Pentagon Press LLP, New Delhi, India for keeping faith with the idea of the book project. Pentagon and its production management have extended excellent support in the process of editorial work. A special thanks to the anonymous reviewers for their detailed, trenchant and yet constructive comments on earlier drafts of the manuscript. We wish to dedicate this book to the millions of people who have suffered from the COVID-19 pandemic. We warmly acknowledge with gratitude the contribution of our friends, colleagues and family members to finish the manuscript in such a short period of time. Finally, we take all responsibility for any errors or omissions whatsoever in the book.

Delwar Hossain
Md. Shariful Islam

1

Introduction

I'm not trying to give either an optimistic or a pessimistic spin on the challenges in facing our deadliest enemy. I'm trying to be realistic. The only way we are going to confront and deal with the ever-present threat of infectious disease is to understand those challenges so that the unthinkable does not become the inevitable (Osterholm 2017: 17).

The International Health Regulations (IHR) Review Committee, an independent panel of 25 experts convened by WHO, cautioned in 2011, 'The world is ill-prepared to respond to a severe influenza pandemic or to any similarly global, sustained and threatening public health emergency' (Cohen 2011). Almost nine years after the publication of the report, the COVID-19 global pandemic poses the greatest challenge to humanity that the world has never faced since the end of World War II. The COVID-19 pandemic has already affected 213 countries and territories in the world. More than ten million people have been infected by COVID-19 while more than 500, 000 people have died from this pandemic. It has created human insecurities to millions of people in the world. South Asian countries have already suffered from this pandemic crisis. India, Pakistan, and Bangladesh lead the curve of COVID-19-infected people in the region. Although the preventive measures of South Asian countries have generally contained the spread and fatalities from COVID-19, it has a profound impact on every sector of human activity ranging from the economic to education. Particularly, livelihoods and public health systems have been worst affected by COVID-19. The talk of New Normal in the post-COVID-19 era gives some sense of understanding the impact of this crisis on South Asia.

In the case of South Asia, we have seen the struggles of doctors and nurses with the increased pace of infections and given the poorly equipped health system in the region, a long queue for food, or even protests for food, the miserable story of millions of workers who walked hundreds of kilometres to reach their homes after losing their source of income. Consequently, COVID-19 has been a major source of acute human insecurity to the South Asian people, especially for the poor. As chapters three and four show, tens of thousands of people have lost their livelihoods which badly affected their human security and their families. The pandemic has triggered health insecurity, food insecurity, and economic insecurity among many others, in South Asia. Against this background, there is a need for a critical study of the implications of COVID-19 for human security in order to fathom the emerging theoretical and policy issues in the region. Thus, this book provides an understanding of the implications of the COVID-19 global pandemic on human security in South Asia. It is an attempt to address the literature gap on a critical and emerging issue called the COVID-19 global pandemic and its implications for human security that South Asia is facing today. Though COVID-19 merits serious attention from medical research, social science research also becomes pertinent to understand the contexts, implications, and policy responses from a social science perspective. In fact, the study becomes important both from theoretical and policy perspectives. Since there is a knowledge gap on the human security in South Asia in general and linking it with COVID-19 in particular, this book fills the existing knowledge gap. From the perspective of policy, the insights of the study would guide policy makers in South Asia in reframing their security policies emphasising on human security.

Understanding COVID-19 Global Pandemic and Human Security

According to the World Health Organisation (2010), 'A pandemic is the worldwide spread of a new disease. An influenza pandemic occurs when a new influenza virus emerges and spreads around the world, and most people do not have immunity'. For instance, the 1918 influenza pandemic killed at least fifty million people around the world in less than a year (McMillen 2016:4). Pandemics have long-term implications for the survivors. Douglas Almond (2006:672) studied the long term effects of the 1918 influenza pandemic on post-1940 Americans and found that there are 'reduced educational attainment, increased rates of physical disability, lower income, lower socioeconomic status, and higher transfer payments' for children born to infected mothers compared with other birth cohorts.

COVID-19, which originated in Wuhan, China, at the end of December 2019, soon spread globally. On 20 January, the Chinese government officially announced the COVID-19 to the world (cited in Fu and Zhu 2020). On March 12, the World Health Organisation declared the novel coronavirus (COVID-19) a pandemic with major public health threat (Fu and Zhu 2020). Every corner of the world has been affected by this pandemic. It has shown the world that it is high time to rethink the health policies we are practising both nationally and globally, and to rethink what our future holds.

Location and context matter in the case of COVID-19. The meaning of COVID-19 would be quite different to a poor South Asian or African compared to a rich American or European. The socio-economic status also determines the extent of vulnerabilities that one faces. In this context, Eleanor Krassen Covan (2020:239), in an editorial in *Health Care for Women International* writes that

> While indoor plumbing is taken for granted by most Americans, my mind wonders to a Nairobi slum where clean water, personal hygiene products, and soap remain in short supply. I also think about villages in Central Vietnam that have no water. Vietnamese Americans told me this is the consequence of a dam built by the Chinese to keep that water for themselves.

Lockdown measures and business closures have been strictly followed by the countries of the world including South Asian countries to contain the spread of COVID-19 which has created human insecurities to South Asian people as the rest of the chapters of the book shows. In fact, the implications of COVID-19 have been multidimensional—factories have been shut down, educational institutions around the world have been closed, borders have been closed, exports and imports have been badly affected globally. Thus, it becomes pertinent to investigate the human security implications of COVID-19 in South Asia. The next section focuses on the conceptual analysis of human security.

Understanding Human Security

> For too long, the concept of security has been shaped by the potential for conflicts between states. For too long, security has been equated with the threats to a country's borders. For too long, nations have sought arms to protect their security. For most people today, a feeling of insecurity arises more from worries about daily life than from the dread of a cataclysmic world event. Job security, income security, health security, environmental security, security from crime—these are the emerging concerns of human security all over the world (UNDP 1994:3).

The above quotation from the UNDP (1994) report underscores the problems in the conventional understanding and practice of security and thus requires a reconceptualisation of the understanding and practice of security given the changing security challenges that the people of the world face. Before going to theorise human security, it becomes pertinent to have a look at the concept of security itself. Although the term 'security' has become a household word in today's world of intense insecurities and violent conflicts, it is one of the most 'contested concepts' in the discourse of International Relations in general, and Security Studies in particular. There is no single definition of security. The meaning depends largely on who is defining it. For instance, if a realist like Stephen M. Walt (1991) defines security, then it is linked to military security, while a critical scholar like Ken Booth (2007, 1991) sees security as 'survival-plus' or linked with 'emancipation'. While there is no consensus on the meaning of 'security', 'most scholars within International Relations work with a definition that involves the alleviation of threats to cherished values' (Williams 2008:1).

Conventionally, security is understood as a state's security or national security defined in terms of military power. Against this backdrop, Richard H. Ullman rightly puts it, 'We are, of course, accustomed to thinking of national security in terms of military threats arising from beyond the borders of one's own country' (Ullman 1983: 133). During the Cold War period, security was traditionally perceived as state security defined as territorial protection from external aggression. It has been related more to nation-states than to people. But the end of the Cold War resulted in a geopolitical turning point from which the concept of human security emerged (Owen 2012).

Additionally, in the early 1990s, the nature of security threats changed from inter-state to intra-state conflicts. Ethnic conflicts, human rights abuses, chronic poverty, hunger, disease, malnutrition became the pervasive phenomenon in the twenty-first century, which also played a role in the emergence of the notion of human security. In this respect, it is pertinent to note that the human security discourse as such dates back to the Human Development Report 1994, published by the United Nations Development Programme (UNDP). In its 1994 UNDP Report, human security is defined from mainly two aspects. According to the report, 'It means, first, safety from such chronic threats as hunger, disease and repression. And second, it means protection from sudden and hurtful disruptions in the patterns of daily life—whether in homes, in jobs or in communities' (UNDP 1994: 23). In addition, human security is about 'freedom from fear' and 'freedom from want' as it was originally described in UNDP report. Consequently, seven major areas have been identified in the domain of Human Security: Economic security, Food security, Health security, Environmental security, Personal security, Community security, Political security. In fact, one can also look back. In 1939, Abraham Epstein, for instance, contended that 'The fact that the people's security today must be promoted by means of economic improvements rather than by means of armies and battleships' (Epstein 1939: 81). This underscores the necessity of human security.

From a policy perspective, the former UN Secretary-General Kofi Annan (2001) provides a broad definition of human security. According to him, 'Human security can no longer be understood in purely military terms. Rather, it must encompass economic development, social justice, environmental protection, democratisation, disarmament, and respect for human rights and the rule of law' (Annan, 2005). Along with freedom from fear and want, 'the freedom of future generations to inherit a healthy environment' has been added by Kofi Annan in the domain of human security.

Theoretically, after 20 years of its publication, the concept of human security and its 'accompanying agenda' are 'still in a state of flux' (Breslin and Christou 2015: 1). However, the Commission on Human Security defines human security as 'to protect the vital core of all human lives in ways that enhance human freedoms and human fulfilment...protecting people from critical (severe) and pervasive (widespread) threats and situations' (2003: 4). For Amartya Sen, 'human security is concerned with reducing and when possible removing the insecurities that plague human lives' (cited in Commission on Human Security 2003: 9). Tadjbakhsh and Chenoy (2008: 71) contend that 'human security should not be given a narrow definition, but should remain flexible enough to develop as our understanding of the roots of worldwide insecurity deepens as does our capacity to address them'. Many view human security as a people-centred approach. For P.B. Fisher (2011:296), for instance, 'Human security concerns human wellbeing, and the opportunity and capacity to ensure human life, and the dignity associated with that life'. For Geoffrey D. Dabelko, 'Human security evokes the faces of the world's poor, in rural and urban areas, struggling to earn a living. The name itself places the individual and human wellbeing at centre stage, revealing the insufficiency of a state-based approach to security' (Dabelko 2010: ix).

Considering the above definitions, it can be claimed that human security identifies people as the referent object of security instead of state or governments and focuses on the human development, well-being and dignity of the people and the threats they face to their security. While examining the human security implications of COVID-19 in South Asia, four areas, i.e., health security, food security, economic security, and environmental security have been purposively selected.

This book is divided into eight chapters including Introduction and Conclusion. In the Introduction, the background, and purpose of the study, and the theoretical understanding on the concept of human security has been discussed. The second chapter focuses on the implications of COVID-19 on health security in South Asia. It argues that health security has been neglected in South Asia throughout the decades due to the overarching emphasis on military security. The chapter finds that COVID-19 has severe health security implications in South Asia which merits serious attention. It is also argued that health security matters for sustainable long-term personal, national, and regional development in South Asia. Therefore, the chapter strongly suggests investing in the health sector generously for the long-term benefits of the people of the region.

Chapter three investigates COVID-19 implications on food security in South Asia. It argues that COVID-19 has devastating impacts on the food security of South Asians. Most of the people work in informal sectors in the region. Lockdown measures and business closures in the region created impediments to the movement of commodities to consumers. Thus, the supply chain shock due to the transportation, physical and economic restrictions, and the consequent business closures have created severe unemployment problems, which ultimately affected food security. The chapter also focuses on the policy imperatives for sustainable food security in South Asia in the context of infectious disease like COVID-19.

South Asia faces several challenges of economic security, which include poverty, inequality, and injustice as seen in the everyday life of millions of people. Unemployment, low wages, discrimination, corruption, and rent-seeking continuously loom large in the living conditions of more than ninety five per cent of people. In this context, chapter four investigates the linkage between the COVID-19 crisis and economic security in South Asia. How does COVID-19 influence economic security in South Asia? What might be the possible policy responses to address the COVID-19 implications on South Asian economic security both in short and long terms? This chapter has addressed these questions based on desk review. It argues that South Asia has been severely affected due to the impacts of COVID-19 on different dimensions of the economy—trade, investment, aid and technology. The chapter demonstrates that without due attention to the sources of economic insecurity in South Asia, no sustainable progress can be achieved.

Chapter five focuses on the implications of COVID-19 on environmental security in South Asia with a special reference to air pollution and climate change. Though the COVID-19 global pandemic created some negative consequences for humans, it has been a blessing for the environment especially in the cases of air pollution and climate change. Due to lockdown measures and business closures, there is a significant reduction of carbon emissions, both regionally and globally. Air pollution has been reduced significantly in South Asia. The chapter argues that the COVID-19 global pandemic is a wake-up call to save the global environment from imminent destruction. It becomes of paramount interest to ensure clear air, address global climate change for the sustainable wellbeing of the people in South Asia and beyond. It is also critically important to nurture cognitive awareness for a sustainable planet derived from the COVID-19 global pandemic. Thus, the chapter suggests taking a lesson from COVID-19 and maintaining a healthy balance between corporate profits and the environment.

Chapter six focuses on the role of regional cooperation in promoting and securing South Asian human security against the backdrop of COVID-19. As a global pandemic, the COVID-19 crisis makes a strong case for transnational cooperation. Multilateral initiatives are the imperatives that could contribute to deal with the challenge of COVID-19. Given the existing global trends towards parochialism and xenophobia, many argue that COVID-19 will bring strong nationalism, restrict cooperation, and embrace protectionist policies and measures. Against this backdrop, the chapter argues that it is an inescapable imperative for South Asia to focus on regional cooperation to effectively deal with the multidimensional challenges of COVID-19. The chapter focuses on the role of regional cooperation in promoting and securing South Asian human security in the context of COVID-19.

Chapter seven investigates three questions: What factors have led to the crisis of global health governance in addressing COVID-19 global pandemic? What would be the implications of global health governance crisis for South Asia? What can be done to strengthen global health governance in the post-COVID-19 era? The chapter argues that non-cooperation, crisis of global leadership, marginalisation of the World Health Organisation (WHO), marginalisation of science from policy processes have contributed to the crisis of global health governance. The chapter brings the case of strengthening the World Health Organisation for better global health governance.

Chapter eight focuses on concluding remarks and the way forward. It argues for prioritising health in the global agenda, mainstreaming human security in policy and scholarship, reinforcing regional and global cooperation on health, rebuilding economies, promoting the role of science, and deepening cooperation with China. It is argued that one of the sources of abundance for South Asia is its population. Thus, it becomes important to invest in the South Asian people. In this context, in the policy domain, human security needs to be mainstreamed in South Asia taking the human as the referent object of security instead of national security. It becomes important to take lessons from COVID-19 and thus prioritising human security with a special reference to health security. In this context, the chapter argues that South Asia's weak healthcare infrastructure needs to be reinvigorated. Health needs to be the top-most priority for the region. In this case, a unified region-wide strategy for preparedness and response will be imperative to face any future pandemic/epidemic. Infection prevention and control and disease surveillance also becomes important which requires generous investments in health and regional cooperation.

REFERENCES

Almond, D. (2006). Is the 1918 influenza pandemic over? Longterm effects of in utero influenza exposure in the post-1940 U.S. population. *Journal of Political Economy, 114* (4), 672-712.doi:10.1086/507154

Annan, K.A. (2005). *Towards a culture of peace: Letters to future generations.* http://www.unesco.org/opi2/lettres/TextAnglais/AnnanE.html.

Booth, K. (1991). Security and emancipation. *Review of International Studies, 17* (4) 313-326.

Booth. K. (2007). *Theory of World Security.* New York: Cambridge University Press.

Breslin, S. & Christou, G. (2015). Has the human security agenda come of age? Definitions, discourses and debates. *Contemporary Politics, 21* (1), 1-10.

Cohen, Jon. (2011, March 11). Committee sharply critiques WHO's pandemic response. Retrieved from https://www.sciencemag.org/news/2011/03/committee-sharply-critiques-whos-pandemic-response

Commission on Human Security (2003). *Human security now: Protecting and empowering people.* New York: United Nations.

Dabelko, G.D. (2010). Foreword. In R.A. Matthew, J. Barnett, B. McDonald, and K.L. O'Brien (Eds.), *Global environmental change and human security* (ix-x), Boston: MIT Press.

Epstein, A. (1939). Government's responsibility for economic security. *The Annals of the American Academy of Political and Social Science, 206,* 81-85.

Fisher, P.B. (2011). Climate change and human security in Tuvalu. *Global Change, Peace & Security: formerly Pacifica Review: Peace, Security & Global Change, 23*(3), 293-313, DOI: 10.1080/14781158.2011.601852.

Fu, K. & Zhu, Y. (2020). Did the world overlook the media's early warning of COVID-19?, *Journal of Risk Research,* DOI: 10.1080/13669877.2020.1756380

McMillen, C.W. (2016). *Pandemics: A very short introduction.* New York: Oxford University Press.

Osterholm. M.T. (2017). *Deadliest enemy: Our war against killer germs.* New York: Little Brown and Company.

Owen, T. (2012). Human security: A contested concept. In Burgess, J. Peter (ed.), *The Routledge handbook of new security studies* (pp. 39-49). Abingdon, Oxon: Routledge.

Tadjbakhsh, S. & Chenoy, A.M. (2008). *Human security: Concepts and implications.* Abingdon, Oxon: Routledge.

UNDP (1994). *Human Development Report 1994.* New York: Oxford University Press.

Ullman, R. (1983). Redefining security. *International Security, 8* (1), 129-153.

Walt, S.M. (1991). The renaissance of security studies. *International Studies Quarterly, 35* (2), 211-239.

Williams, P. D. (2008). Security Studies: An Introduction. In P. D. Williams (ed.), *Security Studies: An Introduction,* (pp.1-12), Oxon: Routledge.

World Health Organization. (2010, February 24). What is a pandemic? Retrieved from https://www.who.int/csr/disease/swineflu/frequently_asked_questions/pandemic/en/

2

Health Security in South Asia

ABSTRACT

How does COVID-19 impact health security in South Asia? How can future health insecurity be addressed? This chapter investigates these questions. It argues that health security has been neglected in South Asia through the decades due to the overarching emphasis on military security. The chapter finds that COVID-19 has severe health security implications in South Asia which merit serious attention. It is also argued that health security matters for sustainable long-term personal, national, and regional development in South Asia. Therefore, the chapter strongly suggests investing in the health sector generously for the long-term benefits of the people of the region.

Keywords: *COVID-19, health insecurity, mental health, conflicts, South Asia.*

Introduction

If we look at the importance of health—as a security issue—it is undeniable because health insecurity can change everything, including our plans, goals, dreams, and life. It is important not only at the individual but also at the state level since the outbreak of disease can challenge an individual's survival as well as a nation's existence. Studies (e.g., McNeill 1978, Price-Smith 2002) have revealed how disease can confront societies as well as affect human fate. The recent case of the COVID-19 global pandemic clearly demonstrates this. Health security in South Asia is important and yet understudied. Thus, the chapter addresses the existing knowledge gap. This article uses novel coronavirus (COVID-19) as a health security threat in South Asia. COVID-19 has shown the world that even the most powerful countries in the world become helpless when faced with diseases. Novel coronavirus crisis which started in December 2019 in China has already resulted in about 300,000 deaths and more than four million infected as of May 10, 2020, around the world. Thus, it becomes pertinent to investigate the health (in) security implications of COVID-19 for South Asia. Against this backdrop, the paper investigates: how does COVID-19 influence health security in South Asia? How can health insecurity be addressed in the future?

This chapter is divided into five sections. The first conceptualises health security, while the second discusses the state of health security in South Asia. The third section focuses on the health security implications of COVID-19 in South Asia. The fourth section takes into account the possible policy responses while the final section delves into concluding remarks.

Theorising Health Security

Before going to investigate the state of health security in South Asia, it is pertinent to look at a few questions. What is health? In addition, what is health security? The World Health Organisation (WHO) defines health as 'a state of complete physical, social, and mental well-being and not merely the absence of disease or infirmity' (WHO, n.d.a.). Although the linkage between health and security and peace was recognised in the constitution of the World Health Organisation in 1946 (World Health Organisation 2006), health was a neglected area both in theory and in practice due to the overarching emphasis on military security during the Cold War period. Colin McInnes argues, 'the relationship between health and security has been limited and unidirectional' (McInnes 2008: 275). Following the end of the Cold War, health security came to the forefront in both academic debates as well as practice with the release of the 1994 United Nations Development Programme Report entitled *New Dimensions of Human Security*. Consequently, health has been framed as a security threat by the academic community (Price-Smith 2002; Davies 2008; Yuk-ping and Thomas 2010; 2013; Nunes 2014; McInnes 2015). However, Yuk-ping and Thomas (2010) note that in the security studies discourse, there are very few scholarly works that identify disease as a threat to national or human security and wellbeing. Even Barry Buzan's (1983) *People, States and Fear*, a seminal contribution to the discussion on 'broadening' and 'deepening' security, which includes five sectors of security (military, political, economic, societal, and environmental) overlooks health security.

However, in terms of significance, 'health challenges—whether from infectious disease or biohazards—represent a clear and distinct form of security threat' (Yuk-Ping and Thomas 2013:5-6). For instance, the unprecedented Ebola outbreak in West Africa in 2014-15 caused more than 10,000 deaths and resulted in 'global health security risk' (McInnes 2016). In fact, in this age of globalisation, the Ebola virus infected people who had travelled across borders within Africa, to Europe to North America and Asia. Thus, though the border can be controlled or the movement of people can be restricted under the Westphalian notion of sovereignty, the spread of infectious diseases cannot be similarly controlled. For instance, the outbreak of severe acute respiratory syndrome (SARS) in 2003 reminded the world that border controls could not stop the international spread of disease. Indeed, following the outbreak of SARS, the International Health Regulations of WHO was broadened in scope. Studying health security, therefore, merits serious attention. Concerning the definition of health security, William Aldis notes:

> A search of the term [health security] using an internet search engine confirms an alarming lack of agreement on the meaning and scope of the concept [health security]. Of the first 100 citations found on the search, 44 referred only to bio-terrorism or trans-border spread of disease, 36 referred to effects of rising health care costs and health insurance in developing countries, 2 referred only to HIV/AIDS, 10 referred to unrelated matters (e.g. electronic home protection systems), and only 7 referred to 'health security' in the sense intended by the UNDP (Aldis 2008:372).

Health security has been defined from the perspective of the infectious diseases, HIV and AIDS, and biological weapons/bioterrorism which is of concern to the West (Feldbaum and Lee 2004:22-24, cited in Rushton 2011:782). These definitions of health security take the state as the referent object of security and serve the security interests of the developed world. In addition, the containment of outbreaks of diseases is mostly focused on and prioritised compared to the prevention aspect of the diseases. Against this backdrop of statist approaches to health security, in a short commentary Joao Nunes (2015) argues that:

> Health security pertains to the forms of harm and vulnerability that individuals experience: not only those resulting from or multiplied by disease (like disability or destitution), but also pre-existing vulnerabilities that give rise to disease in the first place (like malnutrition or insufficient knowledge about the causes of disease). Even though an individual's health status obviously depends on the societal context and on conditions that are provided by states (like health systems or sanitation infrastructure), the ultimate referent for thinking about health security in these approaches is the individual.

In the context of South Asia, health security needs to be defined as incorporating a wider range of threats or issues that threaten individual health and well-being. It can be defined as the alleviation of the insecurities to people arising from health challenges like air pollution, growing food adulteration, malnutrition, hunger, and diseases including infectious diseases like COVID-19. It is also alleviating the impediments to the physical and mental growth of an individual. Thus, one can argue that South Asia needs a people-centred understanding of health security based on well-being.

State of Health Security in South Asia

Though South Asia is rising in terms of economic growth, it has not been able to ensure better health for the majority of the people in the region. For instance, Laurie Garrett (2001: 4) contends that 'In India's case, economic progress brought worsening public health. The federal government, eager to spend its growing wealth on nuclear weapons and military efforts, relinquished all responsibility for the health of its one billion citizens'. As a result, 'India had no real national public health infrastructure at the end of the twentieth century: no surveillance system, no reporting mechanism, barely a vital statistics registry' (Garrett 2001:4). The picture is similar for other South Asian countries. The COVID-19 crisis clearly shows the fragile healthcare system in South Asia. Consequently, the number of malnourished people, maternal mortality rates, and infant mortality rates are staggering for the region. More specifically, the number of maternal deaths in South Asia was estimated to be 66,000 in 2015 while newborn deaths amounted to one million (WHO *et al.* 2015; UNICEF 2016). Coming in this twenty-first century, these preventable deaths are unfortunate. In fact, to save the South Asian future, it becomes important to save newborn babies.

There is growing health inequality in societies, and therefore, poor health security prevails in South Asia. Here, the elites in the society can access health services while the majority cannot. South Asia also experienced the deadly outbreak of Swine Flu in 2009 and 2015. In addition, the AIDS epidemic along with other diseases poses a major security threat in the region. It is argued that 'Existing infectious diseases like TB, HIV and malaria have been worsened by emerging ones like dengue, chikungunya, healthcare-associated infections and antimicrobial resistance. The region is also an epicentre of an epidemic of lifestyle diseases' (Nagral and Jafarey 2020). Poor hygiene and sanitation, safe water shortages, weak healthcare infrastructures in the region, and the growing inequalities exacerbate the situation. However, the dominant understanding and practice of security in South Asia are based on the realist paradigm which emphasises state security (Banerjee 2000; Behera 2001; Barthwal-Datta 2012).

Hate and Gannon in their study (2010:1) find that South Asia spends less than 3.2 per cent of its GDP on health while the global average is 8.2, and its expenditure has diminished from 2000 to 2006 (for the details of health statistics, see Table 1). Therefore, poor investment on health sector makes poor healthcare infrastructure.

Table 1 demonstrates that while the global average per capita health expenditure in 2016 was US$ 1,001, it was only US$ 191.25 for South Asia and excluding the Maldives and Sri Lanka the average per capita health

Table 1: Health Statistics in South Asia

Country	Life Expectancy at Birth	Current Health Expenditure (CHE) per capita (US$)	CHE as percentage of GDP	Under-five mortality rate (per 1000 live births)	Neonatal mortality rate (per 1000 live births)
	2016	2016	2016	2017	2017
Afghanistan	Male=61.0 Female=64.5 Both sexes=62.6	57	10.2	Male=72 Female=64 Both sexes=68	39
Bangladesh	Male=71.1 Female=74.4 Both sexes=72.7	34	2.4	Male=35 Female=30 Both sexes=32	18
Bhutan	Male=70.4 Female=70.8 Both sexes=70.6	91	3.5	Male=34 Female=28 Both sexes=31	17
India	Male=67.4 Female=70.3 Both Sexes=68.8	62	3.6	Male=39 Female=40 Both Sexes=39	24
Maldives	Male=77.2 Female=79.9 Both Sexes=78.4	1048	10.6	Male=9 Female=7 Both Sexes=8	5
Nepal	Male=68.8 Female=71.6 Both Sexes=70.2	45	6.3	Male=36 Female=31 Both Sexes=34	21
Pakistan	Male=65.7 Female=67.4 Both Sexes=66.5	40	2.8	Male=78 Female=71 Both Sexes=75	44
Sri Lanka	Male=72.1 Female=78.5 Both Sexes=75.3	153	3.9	Male=10 Female=8 Both Sexes=9	6

Source: WHO (2019:80-87).

expenditure for the remaining six South Asian countries stand at the only US$ 54.83. The Table also shows that Bangladesh invests the lowest in South Asia, only 2.4 per cent of its GDP while Maldives spends most, 10.6 percent of its GDP on health. In the case of India, for instance, Shukla (2020) writes that 'there is no alternative to infusing much higher level of resources into public health systems. This involves increasing public health budgets substantially, at least to achieve the National Health Policy goal of elevating public health spending to 2.5 per cent of the GDP by

2025 (currently it hovers around just 1.2 per cent)'.) Consequently, in the indicators of life expectancy, under-five mortality rate or neonatal mortality rate, Maldives is doing great in South Asia. For instance, in the context of neonatal mortality rate (per 1000 live births), the lowest mortality rate is in the Maldives: only five while Pakistan stands highest estimating 44. Table 1 also tells us that under-five or neonatal mortality rate works as a major health challenge in South Asia. According to the World Bank, in Afghanistan, about one in every 10 children die before reaching the age of five, and there are about 396 deaths per every 100,000 births while the 2015 world average was 216 (cited in *Al Jazeera* 2016). Since South Asian countries invest less in the healthcare sector, the healthcare infrastructure is very weak (Tables 2 and 3).

Table 2: Medical Doctors (per 10,000 population) (2001-2018)

Year	Afghanistan	Bangladesh	Bhutan	India	Maldives	Nepal	Pakistan	Sri Lanka
2001	1.9	2.5		5.37			6.59	4.43
2002		-		5.55				-
2003		2.71		5.63				-
2004		2.81	1.85	5.72	9.7	2.12	7.42	5.41
2005		3.08		5.76			7.88	5.22
2006	1.6	3.17		5.85				5.22
2007	1.74	3.29	2.17	5.98	16.47		7.62	5.56
2008	1.74	3.42	2.55	6.14			7.81	6.24
2009	2.13	3.54		6.22	14.88		7.95	6.83
2010	2.37	3.64		6.62	14.36		8.08	7.24
2011	2.52	3.84		7.38			8.31	7.39
2012	2.41	4	2.77	6.98		5.16	8.59	7.65
2013	2.85	4.22	2.86	-		5.64	8.77	7.98
2014	2.98	4.89	3.39	7.25	17.7		8.97	8.36
2015	2.85	4.86	3.45	-	28.86		9.26	8.62
2016	2.78	4.97	4.06	7.59			9.62	8.93
2017		5.43	4.02	7.78	37.23	9.1	10.01	9.28
2018		5.81	4.24	8.57	45.63	7.49	9.8	10.04

Source: WHO (n.d.b).

Tables 2 and 3 clearly demonstrate how poor South Asian healthcare infrastructure is. For instance, in Afghanistan, there were only 2.78 medical doctors for 10,000 people in 2016. There were 5 hospital beds for 10,000 people in 2015. Only one bed increased between 2006 and 2015. In fact, decades of war and poverty have made the Afghanistan healthcare system weak (Latifi 2019). Abdullah said, 'With what we spend on a single day of war, we could build a state-of-the-art hospital' (cited in Latifi 2019). Moreover, healthcare facilities in Afghanistan have been constantly under attack by the armed groups. According to the WHO, in the first quarter of 2019, there were 34 reported attacks which killed at least nine workers and patients and resulted in the closure of 87 medical facilities (cited in Latifi 2019).

Table 3: Hospital Beds per 10, 000 Population (2006-2015)

Country	2006	2007	2008	2009	2010	2011	2012	2013	2014	2015
Afghanistan	4	4	4	4	4	4	5	5	5	5
Bangladesh									6	8
Bhutan										
India						7				
Maldives				43						
Nepal								3		
Pakistan	13	10	6	6	6	6	6	6	6	6
Sri Lanka					35					

Source: WHO (n.d.c.).

For Nepal, there were only three hospital bed allocated for 10, 000 people in 2012. This makes the scarcity of hospital beds in South Asia. Even many new-born babies do not get a bed in government hospitals in South Asia. This poor healthcare impedes the drastic reduction of the maternal and neonatal mortality ratio. Consequently, maternal mortality still works as a major challenge in the case of health security in South Asia. One needs to look at Table 4, to understand the maternal mortality ratio in South Asia.

Table 4 shows that though the ratio of maternal mortality has been reduced significantly for some countries, it is still high for other countries in South Asia which can be turned into zero (Table 4) if the healthcare sector is properly taken care of. For Afghanistan, the ratio is still high. From Table 4, one can imagine how many mothers have died in South Asia over the decades. In fact, neonatal or maternal mortality depends on several factors. Among the factors, the presence of skilled health personnel during birth becomes important. It becomes pertinent to have a look at Table 5 to understand the trends of skilled health personnel attendance during birth.

Table 4: Maternal Mortality Ratio (per 100,000 live births) (2002-2015)

Year	Afghanistan	Bangladesh	Bhutan	India	Maldives	Nepal	Pakistan	Sri Lanka
2002	1300	410		336	105	520	264	50
2003	1240	395		319	97	470	254	50
2004	1180	372		303	89	447	243	48
2005	1140	343		286	75	415	237	45
2006	1120	315		270	71	386	222	47
2007	1090	297		255	71	361	214	43
2008	1030	280		240	72	342	205	42
2009	993	269		225	71	323	199	41
2010	954	258		210	67	305	191	38
2011	905	248		197	62	285	180	38
2012	858	238		185	60	266	173	37
2013	810	227		175	58	248	166	37
2014	786	214		166	56	231	161	36
2015	701	200		158	54	236	154	36

Source: WHO (n.d.c.).

Table 5: Births Attended by Skilled Health Personnel (%) (2002-2015)

Year	Afghanistan	Bangladesh	Bhutan	India	Maldives	Nepal	Pakistan	Sri Lanka
2002	-	-	-	-	-	-	23	-
2003	14	14	-	-	-	-	-	-
2004	-	-	-	-	85	-	-	-
2005	-	-	-	-	92	-	31	-
2006	-	20	-	47	94	19	-	-
2007	-	18	-	-	96	-	36	99
2008	-	-	-	52	98	-	-	-
2009	-	-	-	-	97	-	41	-
2010	34	27	-	-	98	-	-	-
2011	39	32	-	-	99	36	43	-
2012	40	-	-	-	96	-	51	-
2013	-	34	-	-	96	-	55	-
2014	45	42	-	81	96	56	-	-
2015	51	-	-	-	-	-	-	-

Source: WHO (n.d.c.).

Though data on births attended by skilled health personnel is not available for many years for most of the countries in South Asia, available data in Table 5 demonstrates that, in overall, the picture is not satisfactory. Except for the Maldives and Sri Lanka, the percentage of skilled health personnel attendance during birth is very disappointing. The makes the number of maternal mortality and neonatal mortality high. Among the major reasons, the socio-economic conditions of the South Asian people, growing health inequalities, income inequalities, insufficient skilled health personnel especially in the rural areas, and the rising cost of health care as a result of privatisation of healthcare are primarily responsible. The following section discusses the growing privatisation of healthcare systems in South Asia.

Privatisation of Healthcare and Growing Inequalities

Privatisation of healthcare means commercialisation and marketisation of healthcare services by non-state actors. Growing privatisation of healthcare in South Asia since the 1980s and 1990s has been a concern for the poor in the region. In fact, the structural adjustment programme of the World Bank and IMF in the 1980s and 1990s was imperative in the promotion of privatisation of both industrial and services sectors including the health sector. Thus, 'for profit' institutions as a form of private medical colleges, hospitals, and clinics were accelerated and funded by non-state actors in South Asia. In this twenty-first century, business in the health sector has been good in the region. The vast majority of the people in the region, i.e., the poor, cannot afford the high cost of private medical services. For instance, in the case of Bangladesh, the *New Age* (March 9, 2019) reports that 'Deviating from the approved chart for medical services, they (private hospitals, clinics) usually charge between Tk 15,000 (US$ 177) and Tk 30,000 (US$ 353) for a minor surgery like appendectomy or delivery while reputed hospitals such as Square Hospital charge about Tk 125,000 (US$ 1471) for a minor surgery. The higher out-of-pocket public health expenditure in Bangladesh is indicative of (the) ethically compromised practice of health service providers'. Additionally, due to the poor healthcare infrastructure in the public health system in the region, the people (who can afford, i.e., the rich) prefer private healthcare for treatment with high costs. It becomes a daunting task for tens of thousands of poor people in the region to bear the rising costs of medicare. Abhay Shukla (2020) writes in *Indian Express* that the private sector provides over 70 per cent of healthcare in India. In the case of privatisation of healthcare in India, Shukla (2020) notes that:

> Data for last two years shows that in the Union Health budget, the share of National Health Mission (dealing mostly with public health services at primary and secondary levels) has dropped from 56 to 49 per cent, while the share of health insurance schemes has risen from 4 to 9 per cent. [W]e might question the recent Niti Aayog proposal to hand over large District hospitals to private operators in PPP mode, shifting these hospitals out of direct public control. Further, these key public facilities would mostly start charging half of their patients at commercial rates. Such privatisation would weaken public health capacities, while fragmenting coordination across levels of care, and increasing the probability of denial of care to those unable to afford, in situations like the emerging scenario when services would be needed the most.

Rampant privatisation of the healthcare sector in Nepal is counterproductive for the vast majority of the people in the country. It is noted that in 1990, there were only 16 private hospitals in Nepal which accelerated to 301 in 2014 (Gurung and Gauld 2014). Notably, 60 per cent of Nepal's doctors work in the private sector while the sector holds two-thirds of hospital beds. Out-of-pocket spending on health in Nepal accounts for 55 per cent of the total health expenditure (Gurung and Gauld 2014). In the case of Pakistan, *Dawn* in its editorial (April 12, 2019) shows how education and health have been neglected in Pakistan. Shehla Zaidi (2019) writes in *Dawn* that:

> 70 per cent of Pakistan's population (66pc rural and 76pc urban), including many from the lower socioeconomic segments, go to private medical providers for routine consultations. 73pc of treatment for diarrhoea in children (the second highest cause of child mortality), 57pc of pregnancy care visits, and 69pc of all births take place in private clinics. The private sector also boasts a substantial share of blood bank, routine laboratory and X-ray services, and in some provinces, ambulance services too.

In addition, there is a growing health inequality in society. Good doctors, nurses, hospitals are available in the urban areas/major (district level) cities. Thus, people in rural areas are deprived of proper healthcare services. On the other hand, there is the rising cost of healthcare due to privatisation and increasing the price of medicines. Thus, the poor section in society is badly affected due to health challenges in South Asia. The COVID-19 global pandemic has worsened the already bad situation of healthcare.

COVID-19 and Vulnerability of South Asian Health System

What are the specific sectors of the health system exposed as vulnerable to COVID-19 as a pandemic and how are they related to the overall health system in South Asia? COVID-19 shows that South Asian countries are ill-equipped to fight diseases like coronavirus. Lack of essential medical equipment including PPE (personal protection equipment) for doctors, and nurses, insufficient ventilators, testing kits, masks for the people, lack of ICU was noted in the fight against COVID-19 in South Asia (Kakar 2020, Singh et al. 2020, *Al Jazeera*, April 4, 2020). In the fight against COVID-19 in India, Abhay Shukla (2020) writes that 'The existing capacities of public hospitals will be massively overstretched since many district hospitals do not have the required facilities due to neglect of public health services in many states'. Ironically, due to lack of PPE and testing kits, COVID-19 has created panic among many healthcare professionals. In Bangladesh for instance, doctors preferred to sit in their chambers and clinics, for a few weeks which resulted in the deaths of many people due to lack of treatment. The ill-equipped health system in South Asia in the fight against COVID-19 resulted in a large number of cases and fatalities (Table 6).

Table 6: Number of Affected and Deaths in South Asia from COVID-19 (As of June 28, 2020)

Country	Number of Affected	Number of Deaths
Afghanistan	30,616	703
Bangladesh	133,978	1,695
Bhutan	75	-
India	529,577	16,103
Maldives	2,305	8
Nepal	12,309	28
Pakistan	198,883	4,035
Sri Lanka	2,033	11

Source: Worldometer (2020). https://www.worldometers.info/coronavirus/#countries

Table 6 shows that the number of affected people and deaths in India, Pakistan and Bangladesh is high. Bhutan is in a better position with only 75 infected while the number of death is zero. It is also important to note that Maldives and Sri Lanka are in a better position in terms of deaths. One can link the lower number of deaths with the better health care infrastructure. As Table 1 demonstrates, Maldives and Sri Lanka invest a substantial amount in the health sector compared to other South Asian countries. Except Bhutan, Maldives, and Sri Lanka other South Asian countries are struggling to fight against COVID-19.

In the case of investing health security in South Asia, it can also be argued that military security has been prioritised at the expense of health security. For instance, between 1990 and 2010, military spending rose from 43 per cent to 388 per cent in South Asia while Europe and Central Asia saw it decline to 69 per cent (UNDP 2013:40). This is because the dominant understanding and practice of security in South Asia are based on the realist paradigm which emphasises state security (Banerjee 2000; Behera 2001; Barthwal-Datta 2012, Islam 2015). However, the critical question is whether human beings die only from war? Do they not die from hunger, malnutrition, and disease? The next section explains COVID-19 as a health security threat in South Asia, which is understudied and thus merits serious attention.

Implications of COVID-19 in South Asian Health Security

South Asia is one of the densely-populated regions in the world. On the one hand, the poor socio-economy condition of people in the region increases vulnerability to infectious diseases like COVID-19 as insufficient access to nutrition lowers immunity. On the other hand, the crowded spaces where tens of thousands of South Asians live makes it easier for any infectious disease to spread. COVID-19 will have health security implications for South Asian people in multiple ways. It is a health security issue in South Asia, considering the enormous loss of lives it caused regionally (Table 6). It is noticed that when a member is affected in a family, other members are also affected. And if the dead person becomes the only earning member of the family, it creates a serious threat to health security, food security, and economic security of other members of the family.

Affecting the General Patients

General patients are severely affected due to the COVID-19 global pandemic. In fact, many doctors were reluctant to see general patients at the beginning of the coronavirus outbreak due to the shortage of PPE for them. Even when the doctors are well-equipped with PPE, they fear to see patients with the corona symptom, i.e., respiratory issues, especially breathing problems. It is reported that on May 9, 2020, an additional secretary of Bangladesh, whose daughter is also a doctor, was denied admission by several hospitals due to his breathing problem and they suggested admission in a special COVID-19 hospital. But the patient's medical history says he was suffering from a kidney problem. When he was taken to the COVID-19 special hospital, he was dead. According to his daughter, her father was dead because of the corona fear and thus negligence of the hospitals (*Samakal*, May 9, 2020). The situation is similar in India. It is reported that there are many cases where general patients are not being admitted or treated in India due to the fear of corona.. As a result, many general patients died due to a lack of treatment (Ghosh 2020). Ghosh notes that there are statistics on the number of deaths from coronavirus but nobody is counting the number of deaths from lack of treatment (Ghosh 2020).

It also becomes a concern when healthcare professionals, including doctors and nurses, are being infected which even resulted in deaths (*Ananda Bazar Patrika*, April 27, 2020; Mahmud 2020). The picture is quite worrying for Bangladesh where more than 300 doctors have been infected with two of them succumbing as on May 4, 2020. When any doctor or nurse becomes infected by COVID-19, other colleagues are quarantined and it is seen that even the whole hospital or wards have been locked down. Thus, general patients are being affected due to the shortage of doctors and nurses. For instance, in Habiganj district, Sylhet, Bangladesh, 16 doctors and nurses were infected by COVID-19. Thus, Habiganj Sadar

Hospital, Chunarughat, and Lakhai health complex have been shut down. Consequently, 800, 000 people are being deprived of treatment due to the closure of these three government hospitals (Das 2020). In fact, the government hospital is the only hope for the tens of thousands of poor and marginalised people in Bangladesh along with other South Asian countries.

Lockdown measures also disrupt the transport system. Many general patients have died due to lack of treatment as they could not reach hospitals due to lockdown, which created a shortage of ambulances. For instance, a Dhaka University student who was not corona infected had some health issues which required regular health checkups. But due to lockdown measures, he could not see the doctor, which resulted in his death. Along with other general patients, many pregnant women have died in South Asia due to lack of treatment and lack of transportation as doctors, hospitals and nurses are busy with corona patients. Also, due to lack of personal protective equipment, doctors are apathetic to treat general patients given the considerable amount of corona fear. Thus, general patients are deprived of proper treatment that influences their health security seriously.

Diverting Critical Resources to Fight COVID-19
The socio-economic condition of South Asian states is poor where the healthcare system is fragile/strained. In this chapter, it is found that while military security becomes prioritised in the policy formulations and execution, health security becomes neglected. Thus, the insufficient budget on the health sector makes the case worse when critical resources are diverted to fight infectious diseases like novel coronavirus. While millions of dollars are invested in fighting COVID-19 in South Asia, resource distribution for other health care sectors becomes severely affected, which affects health security in South Asia.

Mental Health Ramifications
There are clear linkages between pandemic and mental health issue, i.e., anxiety of getting infected, loss of livelihood, symptoms of stress, health anxiety, post-traumatic stress, and suicidality (Wheaton et al., 2012;

Wu et al., 2009; Yip et al., 2010). There are also mental health ramifications of the COVID-19 global pandemic (Lee 2020; Liu et al. 2020; Xiang et al. 2020). Against the backdrop of the COVID-19 outbreak in Wuhan, Liu et al. (2020: e17) notes that 'As a result of the rapidly increasing numbers of confirmed cases and deaths, both medical staff and the public have been experiencing psychological problems, including anxiety, depression, and stress'. As COVID-19 has forced many countries into lockdown, it has created mental health problems for many as people are confined to their homes for weeks. Pragya Lodha, a clinical psychologist and the programme director of the Mumbai chapter of MINDS Foundation, claims that the lockdown crisis in India due to COVID-19 has heightened tensions and created severe anxieties among the public (Neurekar 2020). World Vision surveyed the mental health implications of COVID-19 on children and the young from 13 developing states including Bangladesh. In the survey, it is found that 91 per cent of children and youngsters are facing mental problems due to closure of educational institutions, social distancing or isolation, and the rise of poverty in the family created by the COVID-19 global pandemic (*Prothom Alo*, April 29, 2020). The case many in other South Asian countries.

Additionally, how COVID-19 patients were treated by society impacts the mental health of the affected and his/her family members. Deaths or infected from COVID-19 have shown that the families of the victims are socially boycotted. It created mental disorders in many of the affected families. It is also reported that a COVID-19 patient was beaten and made homeless at midnight by the owner of a house in Dhaka, Bangladesh (*Jugantor*, May 7, 2020). In another case, it was reported that due to corona symptoms, a worker was not allowed to enter the home by his wife and children. Later, the patient took shelter in his sister's house where he finally died (Alam 2020). COVID-19 will have severe long term mental health ramifications for the survivors of dead victims. Furthermore, during the lockdown, social isolation, and quarantine, psychological well-being becomes affected badly. This increases domestic violence. The mental health of many workers is likely to be impacted due to the COVID-19 global crisis. 'For white-coat workers, it will be mainly the mental health toll as a result of the high workload during the crisis. For-white collar workers, their mental health will instead suffer from the effects of isolation and quarantine. Finally, for blue-collar workers, job insecurity and loss of income could lead to mental health issues' (Godderis 2020).

Disrupting Regular Immunisation Services

Nearly a quarter (about 4.5 million) of the world's unimmunised or partially immunised children live in South Asia. Among them, about 97 per cent live in Afghanistan, India, and Pakistan. Superstitions prevail among many South Asians regarding vaccination. Najma Hajikhel, 22, a vaccinator at a Basic Health Centre in Sar-e-Kotal village of Mirbachakot district, Afghanistan contends that 'previously, people (Afghans) didn't have a lot of information about vaccinations. Most of them believed in false rumours, such as vaccinations were not necessary or even harmful' (cited in World Bank 2020).

Due to the COVID-19 outbreak, South Asian countries have stopped regular vaccination programmes of children which might lead to another health disaster for the region as warned by the UNICEF. Bangladesh and Nepal have halted their measles and rubella campaigns while Pakistan and Afghanistan have suspended their polio drives since the COVID-19 pandemic (*The Hindu*, April 28, 2020). Jean Gough, director of UNICEF's South Asia office contends that 'While the COVID-19 virus does not appear to make many children seriously ill, the health of hundreds of thousands of children could be impacted by this disruption of regular immunisation services. This is a very serious threat. Early action is key' (cited in *The Hindu*, April 28, 2020). Thus, COVID-19 disrupts the regular immunisation services in South Asia which impact the health security of tens of thousands of children in the region.

Remittances and Health (In)security

When the only earning member of a family dies, the broader human security including the health security of other family members becomes affected. In the case of South Asian expatriates in the Gulf region, the death or sickness or loss of job of the expatriate creates huge suffering to the family members at home. According to the World Bank, remittances sent home by labour migrants are likely to fall 20 per cent as economic activities will be halted due to the coronavirus pandemic (Lindsay 2020). In the case of South Asia, the decline will be more than 20 per cent. World Bank Group President David Malpass claims that 'The ongoing economic recession caused by COVID-19 is taking a severe toll on the ability to send money home and makes it all the more vital that we shorten the time to recovery for advanced economies' (cited in Lindsay 2020). Many labour migrants have already lost their jobs, and their wages are also affected. This consequence will be more severe in the upcoming months. This will impact broader human security including their health security as well as that of their family. According to the World Bank report, 'Migrant remittances provide an economic lifeline to poor households in many countries. A reduction in remittance flows could increase poverty and reduce households' access to much-needed health services' (cited in Lindsay 2020).

COVID-19, Violence and Conflicts

How does health insecurity lead to violence and conflicts? While 8 to 10 per cent of its budget needs to be spent in health security, it is neglected in South Asia which creates health insecurity. This health insecurity can create conflicts between people. If the earning members of the family become affected by diseases like HIV or SARS or coronavirus, then the human security of other members of the family will be threatened which might increase crime. In the context of Papua New Guineans, it is argued that 'The epidemic poses a serious human security threat to Papua New Guineans. The combined effects of a growing epidemic have the potential to further weaken the state's capacity to provide basic services and public goods' (O'keefe 2010: 297).

Diseases like COVID-19 can lead to conflicts in South Asia which can worsen the human security situation in the region. On the one hand, the socio-economic development of South Asian countries is not satisfactory, while on the other, there are growing income inequalities. Thus, the vast majority of the population becomes severely affected due to the rise of diseases. Millions of people in South Asia who work in informal sectors have lost their livelihoods due to the week-long lockdown arising from reducing the spread of COVID-19. As a result, while a vast section of people in society will fail to meet their necessities due to loss of their source of income, it can increase violence, crimes, and conflicts. It is also shown that poor and hungry people have looted government relief in Jamalpur, Bangladesh. Poor people have also demonstrated in different parts of Bangladesh for food (*The Daily Star*, April 20, 2020). In Delhi, the hungry joined a two kilometre-long queue for food in the peak afternoon sun which underscores the acute poverty of the people (Lalwani and Sharma, 2020). It is also worthy to note that people have also committed suicide due to extreme poverty in the lockdown period arising from COVID-19. For instance, a mother who failed to give food to her five children during the lockdown period attempted to commit suicide in Cox's Bazaar, Bangladesh (Alamgir 2020).

There are linkages between COVID-19 and domestic violence. In fact, due to the lockdown measures, domestic violence has increased at an alarming pace around the world. On April 6, 2020, UN Secretary-General António Guterres warned the world about the rising domestic violence against women related to the COVID-19 pandemic outbreak. According to Guterres, 'The combination of economic and social stresses brought on by the pandemic, as well as restrictions on movement, have dramatically increased the numbers of women and girls facing abuse, in almost all countries' (UN News, April 6, 2020). According to the WHO (2020), domestic violence has increased globally since the COVID-19 outbreak began. Reportedly, the National Commission for Women (NCW), has recorded a more than twofold rise in gender-based violence in India related to COVID-19 (Chandra, April 2, 2020).

COVID-19 has shown that the disease can be a potential source of violence and conflict between or among people in South Asia. In addition, if the Bangladesh government and other international organisations are not able to provide basic medical facilities in case of COVID-19 spreading in Rohingya camps, there is the possibility of rising conflicts between the Rohingyas and the local people in Cox's Bazaar, Bangladesh. Thus, health insecurity has the potential to create conflicts between people which impacts broader human security.

Possible Policy Responses

For sustainable health security, South Asian states need to take into account the following policy responses seriously.

Individual as Referent Object of Security

In the case of South Asia, in both policy and scholarship, the state remains the primary referent object of security which needs to be problematised. In fact, in the case of health security in South Asia, individual needs should be the referent object of security addressing human security concerns.

Investing more on Health

It becomes important to increase the budget on health to provide health care services to all. In the case of COVID-19, Shukla (2020) reiterates that 'public health systems are core social institutions in any society. No amount of strategic purchasing or outsourcing to private actors can replace their irreducible role. At the end of the day, it is public health services which will stand by our side in times of epidemics, and we must give highest priority to strengthening them'. In This chapter, it is found that privatisation of healthcare also works as a major challenge for poor people to access healthcare. Hence, it is imperative to focus on increasing public healthcare services. In fact, COVID-19 has shown that South Asia needs more doctors, ventilators, and ambulances compared to soldiers, tanks, and guns. Public health infrastructure in South Asia needs to be resilient so that in the face of any pandemic, it does not collapse.

Improving Disease Surveillance Systems in Humans and Animals

In this inter-dependent and inter-connected world, any region can be affected by any pandemic/epidemic irrespective of the origin of the disease. Thus, to address future pandemics, there is no alternative but to develop disease surveillance systems in humans and animals in South Asia. In this regard, more investments need to be ensured in medical science research and technology. At airports, land borders, and ports, medical screening/checkups need to be ensured.

Addressing Inequalities

Due to the rising healthcare costs on the one hand, and growing income inequalities, on the other, the poor in society cannot ensure adequate healthcare services in South Asia. Rama V. Baru (2003) shows that privatisation of healthcare in South Asia works as a challenge to ensure health services of/for the large section of poor people. Thus, it is important to keep the cost of healthcare within the reach of the poor in the region. Besides, income inequality needs to be addressed by creating employment opportunities for the poor sections of society. Mothers' education needs to be ensured to promote the health security of the children in general and female children in particular in the rural areas of South Asia including Bangladesh and India. The loss of jobs due to COVID-19 needs to be addressed by the state with the highest priority. In this case, the role of non-state actors also becomes important.

Role of Non-state Actors

State machinery alone cannot ensure health security in the region. Since health challenge matters to everyone, alongside state, non-state actors need to come forward. Notably, community clinics and community-based volunteers are working to improve maternal, new-born, and child healthcare services in rural areas. In addition, different NGOs like BRAC are working to ensure healthcare in the rural areas of Bangladesh though, in the fight against COVID-19, the role of BRAC has been minimal. Civil society organisations (CSOs) including the media, played a crucial role to raise awareness regarding COVID-19 in South Asia. Additionally, though at a minimal level, individuals, NGOs, banks came forward to address the COVID-19 global pandemic in South Asia. This needs to be expanded.

Focusing on Diplomacy

When states focus on war or war-centric understanding, they prioritise military security over anything else. And due to the overemphasis on military security, following the logic of anarchy, health security has been neglected through decades in the region as discussed earlier. Thus, it is important to focus on diplomacy to resolve bilateral disputes and hence invest more in people in South Asia while addressing health insecurities. Concerted efforts using diplomacy to fight any future global pandemic will be necessary.

Role of Individuals

Jonathan S. Abramowitz (2019:xii) contends that 'our behaviour increases the chances of a pandemic'. In addressing the COVID-19 crisis, it is manifested that though some quarters of people cooperated well, many did not cooperate with the government. They hardly cared about social distancing and thus arranged religious gatherings, gatherings at tea stalls, and other social gatherings. Bangladesh, India, and Pakistan are mostly sufferers in the COVID-19 crisis. In this case, the irresponsible behaviour of many individuals is one of the major reasons. In future, public education on infectious diseases needs to be promoted and thus taken into account by policymakers.

Role of Scholars and Scholarship

In the case of South Asia, the role of scholars and scholarship on security studies needs to be problematised. Security Studies in South Asia are mostly dominated by a realist understanding of state/military security. As Cox said, 'theory is always for someone, for some purposes'. IR scholars in general and Security Studies scholars in particular need to rethink their research interest bring a normative understanding. Additionally, Security Studies curricula in South Asia need to be redesigned incorporating critical security studies issues like health security.

Conclusion

This chapter found that health security of the people of South Asia, especially the poor, is badly affected due to the COVID-19 global pandemic. It argues that the dominant understanding of Security Studies in South Asia based on the realist (statist) paradigm needs to be problematised. The individual needs to be the central focus of analysis regarding Security Studies in the region. Due to the dominance of military security in the region, the health security of the people becomes neglected. Thus, the people cannot explore and exploit its fullest potential. COVID-19 affects everyone, whether poor or rich, powerless or powerful in the region. For a bright and sustainable future of the region, there is no alternative except a healthy region. Thus, all the stakeholders concerned, both state and non-state actors, need to come forward to address the health challenges. This chapter concludes by saying that for the betterment and well-being of the people of the region, health security needs to be prioritised in the domain of Security Studies in South Asia, both in policy and theory. Therefore, the states of the region need to invest more in the health of their people. Accelerating regional cooperation on health also becomes important in the face of any future pandemic.

REFERENCES

Abramowitz, J. S. (2019). Foreword. In S. Taylor, *The psychology of pandemics: Preparing for the next global outbreak of infectious disease* (xi-xiii). Newcastle, UK: Cambridge Scholars Publishing.

Aldis, W. (2008). Health security as a public health concept: a critical analysis. *Health Policy and Planning, 23,* 369–375.

Alamgir, S. (2020, April 13). Mother attempted to commit suicide as failed to provide food to children [In Bangla]. *Daily Ittefaq.* Retrieved from https://www.ittefaq.com.bd/wholecountry/144444/%E0%A6%B8%E0%A6%A8%E0%A7%8D%E0%A6%A4%E0%A6%BE%E0%A6%A8%E0%A6%A6%E0%A7%87%E0%A6%B0-%E0%A6%96%E0%A6%BE%E0%A6%AC%E0%A6%BE%E0%A6%B0-%E0%A6%A6%E0%A6%BF%E0%A6%A4%E0%A7%87-%E0%A6%A8%E0%A6%BE-%E0%A6%AA%E0%A7%87%E0%A6%B0%E0%A7%87-%E0%A6%AE%E0%A6%BE%E0%A7%9F%E0%A7%87%E0%A6%B0-%E0%A6%86%E0%A6%A4%E0%A7%8D%E0%A6%AE%E0%A6%B9%E0%A6%A4%E0%A7%8D%E0%A6%AF%E0%A6%BE%E0%A6%B0-%E0%A6%9A%E0%A7%87%E0%A6%B7%E0%A7%8D%E0%A6%9F%E0%A6%BE-%C2%A0?fbclid=IwAR0bEaL1U5JzEGxtg07zRFH0KTSxizcZ1xroz1SujVF3QPTYu2aDEsqaz3g

Al Jazeera (2016, August 10). Afghanistan's healthcare system struggles to rebound. Retrieved from https://www.aljazeera.com/news/2016/08/afghanistan-health-care-system-struggles-rebound-160810104017464.html

Al Jazeera (2020, April 4). Pakistan ill-equipped to fight COVID-19: Healthcare workers. Retrieved from https://www.aljazeera.com/news/2020/04/pakistan-ill-equipped-fight-COVID-19-healthcare-workers-200404095933357.html

Alam, M. (2020, May 7). Coronavirus: Was not allowed to enter home by wife, and children and finally worker dies in his sister's house [In Bangla]. *Dhaka Tribune.* Retrieved from https://bangla.dhakatribune.com/bangladesh/2020/05/07/23072/%E0%A6%95%E0%A6%B0%E0%A7%8B%E0%A6%A8%E0%A6%BE%E0%A6%AD%E0%A6%BE%E0%A6%87%E0%A6%B0%E0%A6%BE%E0%A6%B8:-%E0%A6%98%E0%A6%B0%E0%A7%87-%E0%A6%A2%E0%A7%81%E0%A6%95%E0%A6%A4%E0%A7%87-%E0%A6%A6%E0%A7%87%E0%A7%9F%E0%A6%A8%E0%A6%BF-%E0%A6%B8%E0%A7%8D%E0%

A6%A4%E0%A7%8D%E0%A6%B0%E0%A7%80-%E0%A6%B8%E0%A6%A8%
E0%A7%8   D%E0%A6%A4%E0%A6%BE%E0%A6%A8%E0%A6%B0%
E0%A6%BE,-%E0%A6%AC%E0%A7%8B%E0%A6%A8%E0%A7%87%
E0%A6%B0-%E0%A6%AC%E0%A6%BE%E0%A7%9C%E0%A6%BF%E0%
A6%A4%E0%A7%87-%E0%A6%B6%E0%A7%8D%E0%A6%B0%E0%A6%
AE%E0% A6% BF%E0%A6%95%E0%A7%87%E0%A6%B0-%E0%A6%AE%
E0%A7%83%E0%A6%A4%E0%A7%8D%E0%A6%AF%E0%A7%81

Ananda Bazar Patrika (2020, April 27). Corona positive doctor dies in West Bengal: 461 are infected at the moment [In Bangla]. Retrieved from https://www.ananda bazar.com/state/coronavirus-in-west-bengal-corona-positive-doctor-died-in-bengal-total-461-active-cases-till-now-1.1142102?utm_source=abp_newsletter &utm_ medium= email&utm_ campaign=DailyMorningBriefing&tqid=gvGv PWkq AEoBnLJb47agsCeiHdTblynadEhTUxYL

Banerjee, D. (Ed.) (2000). *Security Studies in South Asia: Change and challenges*. New Delhi: Manohar Publishers & Distributors.

Barthwal-Datta, M. (2012). *Understanding security practices in South Asia: Securitization theory and the role of non-state actors*. Oxon: Routledge.

Baru, R.V. (2003). Privatisation of health services: A South Asian perspective. *Economic and Political Weekly*, 38 (42), 4433-4437.

Behera, N. C. (Ed.) (2001). *State, people and security: The South Asian context*. New Delhi: Har-Anand Publications.

Buzan, B. (1983). *People, states and fear national security problem in International Relations*, (2nd Edition), Sussex: Wheatsheaf Books Ltd.

Chandra, J. (2020, April 2). COVID-19 lockdown | Rise in domestic violence, police apathy: NCW. *The Hindu*. Retrieved from https://www.thehindu.com/news/national/COVID-19-lockdown-spike-in-domestic-violence-says-ncw/article31238659.ece

Davies, S. (2008). Securitizing infectious disease. *International Affairs*, 84, 295-313

Das, S. (2020, May 1). Three government hospitals are closed, 800,000 people are deprived from treatment [In Bangla]. *Daily Prothom Alo*. Retrieved from https://www.prothomalo.com/bangladesh/article/1653953/ %E0%A6%A4%E0%A6%BF%E0%A6%A8%E0%A6%9F%E0%A6%BF-%E0%A6%B8%E0%A6%B0%E0%A6%95%E0%A6%BE%E0%A6%B0%E0%A6%BF-%E0%A6%B9%E0%A6%BE%E0%A6%B8%E0%A6%AA%E0%A6%BE%E0%A6%A4%E0%A6%BE%E0%A6%B2-%E0%A6%AC%E0%A6%A8%E0%A7%8D%E0%A6%A7-%E0%A6%B8%E0% A7%87 %E0%A6%AC%E0%A6%BE%E0%A6%AC%E0%A6%9E%E0%A7%8 D%E0%A6%9A%E0%A6%BF%E0%A6%A4-%E0%A6%86%E0%A6%9F-%E0%A6%B2%E0%A6%BE%E0%A6%96

Dawn editorial. (2019, April 12). Tale of neglect. Retrieved from https://www.dawn.com/news/1475591

Garrett, L. (2001). *Betrayal of trust: The collapse of global public health*. New York: Oxford University Press.

Godderis, L. (2020, April 28). The COVID-19 crisis may lead to mental health issues for many workers. International Labour Organization. Retrieved from https://iloblog.org/2020/04/28/the-COVID-19-crisis-may-lead-to-mental-health-issues-for-many-workers/

Ghosh, S. (2020, April 30). Corona fear: Deaths due to lack of treatment [In Bangla]. DW. Retrieved from https://www.dw.com/bn/%E0%A6%95%E0%A6% B0%

E0%A7%8B%E0%A6%A8%E0%A6%BE-%E0%A6%86%E0% A6% A4%E0% A6%99% E0%A7%8D%E0%A6%95-%E0%A6%AC%E0%A6%BF% E0% A6% A8%E0%A6%BE-%E0%A6%9A%E0%A6%BF%E0%A6%95%E0% A6%BF% E0%A7%8E%E0%A6%B8%E0%A6%BE%E0%A7%9F-%E0%A6%AE% E0% A7%83%E0%A6%A4%E0%A7%8D%E0%A6%AF%E0%A7%81/a-53289878? fbclid=IwAR37otnPOqH6—0baA4CD1lhHw_-IadfbfgtKQwz3g3Zb-yvL8Hoqw1QIbc

Gurung, G. & Gauld, R. (2014, September 30). Private gain, public pain: does a booming private healthcare industry in Nepal benefit its people? *British Medical Journal.* Retrieved from https://blogs.bmj.com/bmj/2016/09/30/does-a-booming-private-healthcare-industry-in-nepal-benefit-its-people/

Hate, V., & Gannon, S. (2010). *Public health in South Asia*, Washington: CSIS.

Islam, M.S. (2015). Mapping security for Bangladesh: An emancipatory approach. *Journal of South Asian Studies, 3* (2), 243-260.

Jugantor (2020, May 7). Corona affected patient was beaten and made homeless at midnight by the owner of the house [In Bangla]. Retrieved from https://www.jugantor.com/COVID-19/304922/%E0%A6%AE%E0%A6%A7%E0% A7%8 D%E0%A6%AF%E0%A6%B0%E0%A6%BE%E0%A6%A4%E0%A7%87- %E0%A6%95%E0%A6%B0%E0%A7%8B%E0%A6%A8%E0%A6%BE%E0%A7%9F- %E0%A6%86%E0%A6%95%E0%A7%8D%E0%A6%B0%E0%A6%BE%E0%A6%A8%E0%A7%8D%E0%A6%A4 %E0%A6%AF%E0%A7%81%E0%A6%AC%E0%A6%95%E0%A6%95%E0%A7%87- %E0%A6%AE%E0%A6%BE%E0%A6%B0%E0%A6%A7%E0%A6%B0- %E0%A6%95%E0%A6%B0%E0%A7%87-%E0%A6%A4%E0%A6% BE% E0% A7%9C%E0%A6%BF%E0%A7%9F%E0%A7%87-%E0%A6%A6% E0%A6% BF%E0%A6%B2%E0%A7%87%E0%A6%A8-%E0%A6%AC%E0%A6% BE% E0% A7%9C%E0%A6%BF%E0%A6%93%E0%A7%9F%E0%A6%BE%E0%A6% B2% E0%A6%BE

Kakar, M.A.Z. (2020, April 12). COVID-19 in Afghanistan: Exposing weaknesses in healthcare system. *The Kabul Times.* Retrieved from https://www.the kabultimes.gov.af/2020/04/12/COVID-19-in-afghanistan-exposing-weaknesses-in-healthcare-system/

Lalwani, V. and Sharma, S. (2020, April 18). Watch: In Delhi, hungry people join a 2-km-long food queue in peak afternoon sun. Scroll.in. Retrieved from https://scroll.in/article/959565/watch-in-delhi-hungry-people-join-a-2-km-long-food-queue-in-peak-afternoon-sun

Latifi, A. M. (2019, May 25). Years of war and poverty take toll on Afghanistan's healthcare. *Al Jazeera.* Retrieved from https://www.aljazeera.com/news/2019/05/years-war-poverty-toll-afghanistan-healthcare-190525101842119.html

Lee, S. A. (2020). Coronavirus anxiety scale: A brief mental health screener for COVID-19 related anxiety. *Death Studies,* DOI: 10.1080/07481187.2020.1748481

Lindsay, F. (2020, April 22). World Bank: Global remittances set to decline sharply as a result of coronavirus. *Forbes.* Retrieved from https://www.forbes.com/sites/freylindsay/2020/04/22/world-bank-global-remittances-set-to-decline-sharply-as-a-result-of-coronavirus/#3fad851a60ab

Liu, S., Yang, L., Zhang, C., Xiang, Y., Liu, Z., Hu, S., & Zhang, B. (2020). Online mental health services in China during the COVID-19 outbreak. *The Lancet* Psychiatry, 7(4), e17–e18. https://doi.org/10.1016/S2215-0366(20)30077-8

Mahmud, F. (2020, April 24). Hundreds of doctors in Bangladesh infected with coronavirus. Al Jazeera. Retrieved from https://www.aljazeera.com/news/2020/04/hundreds-doctors-bangladesh-infected-coronavirus-200423080515266.html

McNeill, W. H. (1978). *Plagues and peoples*. New York: Anchor Books.

McInnes, C. (2008). Health. In P. D. Williams (Ed.), *Security Studies: An introduction* (pp. 274-287), Oxon: Routledge.

— (2015). The many meanings of health security. In S. Rushton & J. Youde (Eds.) *Routledge handbook of global health security* (pp. 7-17) Oxon: Routledge.

— (2016). Crisis! What crisis? Global health and the 2014-15 West African Ebola outbreak. *Third World Quarterly*, 37 (3), 380-400.

Nagral, S. & Jafarey, A. (2020, April 29). A task for South Asia. *The Hindu*. Retrieved from https://www.thehindu.com/opinion/op-ed/a-task-for-south-asia/article31457045.ece

Neurekar, M. (2020, April 15). Coronavirus: As mental health services move online, problems of access and privacy emerge. Scroll.in. Retrieved from https://scroll.in/article/957543/coronavirus-as-mental-health-services-move-online-problems-of-access-and-privacy-emerge

New Age (2019, March 9). Perils of unregulated health sector privatisation. Retrieved from https://www.newagebd.net/article/66836/perils-of-unregulated-health-sector-privatisation

Nunes, J. (2014). *Security, emancipation and the politics of health* .Oxon: Routledge.

— 2015, July 9). Is disease a threat to international security. International Relations and Security Network (ISN), ETH Zurich.

O'keefe, M. (2010). HIV and security in Papua New Guinea: National and human insecurity. In V. Luker & S. Dinnen (Eds.), *Civic insecurity: Law, order, and HIV in Papua New Guinea* (pp. 287-301), ANU E Press. Retrieved from https://www.jstor.org/stable/j.ctt24h9kk.24

Price-Smith, A. T. (2002). *The health of nations: Infectious disease, environmental change, and their effects on national security and development*. Cambridge, Massachusetts: The MIT Press.

Prothom Alo (2020, April 29). Education disrupted, 91 percent children and young stars are mentally disturbed [In Bangla]. Retrieved from https://www.prothomalo.com/bangladesh/article/1653637/%E0%A6%95%E0%A6%B0%E0%A7%8B%E0%A6%A8%E0%A6%BE%E0%A7%9F-%E0% A6% B6% E0%A6%BF%E0%A6%95%E0%A7%8D%E0%A6%B7%E0%A6%BE-%E0%A6%AC%E0%A7%8D%E0%A6%AF%E0%A6%BE%E0%A6%B9%E0%A6%A4-%E0%A6%AE%E0%A6%BE%E0%A6%A8%E0%A6%B8%E0%A6%BF%E0%A6%95-%E0%A6%9A%E0%A6%BE%E0%A6%AA%E0%A7%87-%E0% A7% AF% E0%A7%A7-%E0%A6%AD%E0%A6%BE%E0%A6%97-%E0%A6%B6% E0% A6% BF%E0% A6%B6%E0%A7%81%E2%80%93%E0% A6% A4% E0% A6% B0% E0%A7%81%E0%A6% A3?fbclid=IwAR1Thz1zUUAwobazcr3tsLP-QcKp26KkDUwZ9m77SNdJHGdSp4SbAOK4k5Y

Rushton, S. (2011). Global health security: Security for whom? Security from what?', *Political Studies*, 59, 779-796.

Samakal (2020, May 9). Hospital's negligence, additional secretary dies [In Bangla]. Retrieved from https://samakal.com/print/200522365/online

Shukla, A. (2020, March 24). We must give highest priority to strengthening the public health system. *The Indian Express*. Retrieved from https://indianexpress.com/article/opinion/coronavirus-public-health-system-6329470/

Singh, P., Ravi, S. & Chakraborty, S. (2020, March 24). COVID-19: Is India's health infrastructure equipped to handle an epidemic?. Brookings. Retrieved from https://www.brookings.edu/blog/up-front/2020/03/24/is-indias-health-infrastructure-equipped-to-handle-an-epidemic/

The Daily Star (2020, April 20). People demonstrate for food in Savar. Retrieved from https://www.thedailystar.net/coronavirus-update-people-demonstrate-food-in-savar-1894999

The Hindu (2020, April 28). South Asia faces health crisis as children miss vaccination. Retrieved from https://www.thehindu.com/news/international/south-asia-faces-health-crisis-as-children-miss-vaccination/article31457054.ece

UN News (2020, April 6). UN chief calls for domestic violence 'ceasefire' amid 'horrifying global surge'. Retrieved from https://news.un.org/en/story/2020/04/1061052

UNICEF (2016). Reducing newborn mortality in South Asia: A results-based management approach to improving knowledge and accelerating results. Retrieved from https://www.unicef.org/rosa/UNICEF_Newborn_Strategy_2016.compressed.pdf

UNDP (2013). *The rise of the South: Human progress in a diverse world*. Human development report 2013, New York: United Nations Development Programme.

Wheaton, M.G., Abramowitz, J.S., Berman, N.C., Fabricant, L.E., & Olatunji, B.O. (2012). Psychological predictors of anxiety in response to the H1N1 (swine flu) pandemic. *Cognitive Therapy and Research*, 36(3), 210–218.

WHO (n.d.a). Retrieved from http://www.who.int/suggestions/faq/en/

WHO (n.d.b). Retrieved from https://www.who.int/data/gho/data/indicators/indicator-details/GHO/medical-doctors-(per-10-000-population

WHO (n.d.c). Retrieved from https://www.who.int/gho/countries/en/#B

World Health Organization (2006). Constitution of the World Health Organization. *Basic Documents*, Forty-fifth edition, Supplement. Retrieved from: http://www.who.int/governance/eb/who_constitution_en.pdf

WHO, UNICEF, UNFPA, World Bank Group and the United Nations Population Division (2015). Trends in maternal mortality: 1990 to 2015. Retrieved from: https://data.unicef.org/wp-content/uploads/2015/12/Trends-in-MMR-1990-2015_Full-report_243.pdf

WHO (2019). World health statistics 2019: monitoring health for the SDGs, sustainable development goals. Geneva: World Health Organization. Licence: CC BY-NC-SA 3.0 IGO.

World Bank (2020, April 9). Ensuring accessible health care for rural Afghans. Retrieved from https://www.worldbank.org/en/news/feature/2020/04/09/ensuring-closer-health-care-access-to-rural-afghans

Worldometer (2020, May 10). Retrieved from https://www.worldometers.info/coronavirus/#countries

Wu, P., Fang, Y., Guan, Z., Fan, B., Kong, J., Yao, Z., Liu, X., & Hoven, C.W. (2009). The psychological impact of the SARS epidemic on hospital employees in China: Exposure, risk perception, and altruistic acceptance of risk. *Canadian Journal of Psychiatry*, 54, 302–311.

Xiang, Y., Yang, Y., Li, W., Zhang, L., Zhang, Q., Cheung, T., & Ng, C. H. (2020). Timely mental health care for the 2019 novel coronavirus outbreak is urgently needed. *Lancet, 7*, 228–229.

Yip, P. S. F., Cheung, Y. T., Chau, P. H., & Law, Y. W. (2010). The impact of epidemic outbreak: The case of severe acute respiratory syndrome (SARS) and suicide among older adults in Hong Kong. Crisis, 31(2), 86–92.

Yuk-ping, C. L., & Thomas, N. (2010). How is health a security issue? Politics, responses and issues. *Health Policy and Planning, 25*, 447-453.

— (2013). Introduction: Securitizing health. In N. Thomas (Ed.), *Health Security and Governance* (pp. 1-18) Oxon: Routledge.

Zaidi, S. (2019, February 11). Private sector in health. *Dawn*. Retrieved from https://www.dawn.com/news/1463125

3

Food Security in South Asia

ABSTRACT

How does COVID-19 impact on food security in the context of South Asia? What might be the possible policy responses to address food insecurity in South Asia in future? This chapter investigates these questions. It argues that COVID-19 have devastating impacts on the food security of South Asian people. Most of the people work in the informal sectors in the region. Lockdown measures and business closures led to supply chain shock due to the transportation, physical and economic restrictions and business closures have created severe unemployment problems in the region, which ultimately impacted food security. This chapter also focuses on the policy imperatives for sustainable food security in South Asia in the context of infectious diseases like COVID-19.

Keywords: *Food security, South Asia, COVID-19, Poverty, Malnutrition.*

Introduction

'Two months ago no one was really talking about food security, but now it is what everybody is talking about'.
—**Maximo Torero,** Assistant Director-General at the UN Food and Agricultural Organisation (FAO) (cited in *Financial Times*, April 21, 2020).

The above quotation from Torero clearly demonstrates the importance that COVID-19 brings to the subject of food security for the world community. In addition, the headlines of the *Guardian* (May 9, 2020)

'Hundreds queue for food parcels in wealthy Geneva' or the headline of 'Sign of the times: Mile-long line of cars outside California grocery giveaway' in *Reuters* (Nicholson 2020) signals the acute food insecurity even in the developed world that has been created by the novel coronavirus. While poverty, malnutrition, hunger is a common phenomenon in South Asia, the COVID-19 global pandemic worsens the food security situation in the region. From the media reports, it is manifest that people starved, protested, cried, fought, and even committed suicide for food in South Asia due to the consequences of the COVID-19 global pandemic. It is forecast that the world might experience global recession in the post-COVID-19 world which would hit the food security of millions of people in the world in general and South Asia in particular because of the loss of jobs or sources of income, decreased global cooperation on food aid, restricted global trade on food and strong nationalism. In fact, the COVID-19 global pandemic drew the attention of policymakers, scholars, and media on the subject of health, food, and economic security in particular. Against this backdrop, this chapter investigates two questions: How does COVID-19 impact food security in South Asia? What might be the policy imperatives to address food insecurity in South Asia in the context of pandemics?

The chapter is divided into six sections. The first conceptualises food security, while the second focuses on food security in South Asia briefly. The third section discusses the implications of COVID-19 on food security in general. The fourth explains the food security implications of COVID-19 in the context of South Asia. The fifth section focuses on the policy imperatives, and finally, the chapter concludes.

Understanding Food Security

Simply, food security can be defined as a sustainable, secure access of adequate nutritious food at all times and the capability to utilise those foods by individuals, households, and nations. It has been identified as a new security object in the study of Security Studies (Burgess 2012; Wiggings and Slater 2012). Along with environment, energy, cyber, pandemic, and biosecurity, food security 'confronts conventional premises and expectations of status quo security concepts, by suggesting how securitisation processes can shift focus to objects outside of conventional approaches' (Burgess 2012:3). It is argued that food security is 'one of the cornerstones of human existence and 'without [it], other securities are undermined' (Wiggings and Slater 2012:132). Wiggings and Slater (2012:132) contend that 'Food security is about assuring individuals of their capability to lead their lives, by being able to move physically for work and leisure. It also means that as infants and children they were fed well enough to allow development of their physical and mental power'. Shepherd (2012: 196) proposes redefining food security in terms of 'securing vulnerable populations from the structural violence of hunger'. Wiggins and Slater (2012:133) further note that 'Food security is a continuing state: it applies at all times, through life cycles and through seasonal and other temporal variations'.

Dimensions of Food Security

Is food security all about sufficient production in the field and availability in the market? In this respect, P.S. George points out that in the early years, food security implied arrangements for providing the physical supply of an adequate minimum level of food grains for the population in the developing countries during years of normal as well as poor harvests (George 1994:1092). Per Pinstrup-Andersen (2009:5) notes that 'The use of the term food security at the national and global level tends to focus on the supply side of the food equation'. Though one cannot take the supply-side definition of food security, production also matters. In this regard, C. Peter Timmer argues that '[m]ore food does not guarantee greater food security, but increases in local food production clearly help' (Timmer 2015: ix). At the 1974 World Food Conference, food security was defined as: '...availability at all times of adequate world supplies of basic food-stuffs ... to sustain a steady expansion of food consumption ... and to offset fluctuations in production and prices' (cited in Yaro 2004:24). Here the availability of food was emphasised and thus the world invested immensely in the green revolution to increase food production.

However, one needs to problematise the supply side definition of food security as food security is not only about food availability in the market but accessibility, utilisation, and stability of that food. Simon Maxwell contends that 'It has been impossible since the early 1980s to speak credibly of food security as being a problem of food supply, without at least making reference to the importance of access and entitlement' (1996:157). It is, therefore, the Food and Agriculture Organisation of the United Nations that defines food security as 'food security exists when all people, at all times, have physical, social, and economic access to sufficient, safe and nutritious food that meets their dietary needs and food preferences for an active and healthy life' (FAO 2010:8). Hence, all dimensions of food security, i.e., availability, accessibility, nutrition, utilisation, and stability, are essential in the domain of food security conceptualisation where the individual would be the referent object of food security.

Food Security in South Asia: A Brief Account

Food matters, as one cannot survive without food, whether peasant or president. It is an essential need not only for human beings but also for animals and other creatures. However, ensuring food security for the global population has been identified as an 'unprecedented challenge' given the context of 'severely degraded resource base and rising social inequality' (McLachlan & Hamann 2011: 429). In the case of South Asia, on the one hand, the population is increasing. According to data of Worldometers (n.d.), the population of South Asia is estimated at 1,937,285,292 as of May 12, 2020 which is equivalent to 24.89 per cent of the total world population. In terms of population, South Asia is the largest sub-region in Asia. It is projected that in 2030, the population in South Asia will likely be 2,143,126,834. On the other hand, arable land is decreasing due to human settlement, industrialisation, and other material purposes. In addition, there is a growing income inequality. Thus, feeding future South Asian people will be a daunting task, although over the decade, South Asian countries have reduced poverty substantially (Table 1).

Table 1: Number of Poor People in South Asia using 2011 PPP and $1.9/day poverty line

Year	Number of poor (in millions)	Year	Number of poor (in millions)
1981	515.30	2005	509.96
1984	525.30	2008	468.76
1987	531.28	2010	403.71
1990	537.10	2011	331.74
1993	542.79	2012	304.93
1996	519.01	2013	275.38
2002	556.01		

Source: World Bank, http://iresearch.worldbank.org/PovcalNet/povDuplicateWB.aspx

Table 1 demonstrates that while in 1981, the number of poor people in South Asia was 515.30 million; it has been reduced to 275.38 million in 2013. Between 1981 and 2005, the number of poor people has been reduced by 5.34 million only while between 2005 and 2013, it has been reduced by 234.58 million. If one looks at country-wise statistics (Table 2), Maldives, Sri Lanka, and Bhutan have achieved substantial progress where the poverty headcount ratio was less than 2 per cent in 2018. Other countries are also doing better in terms of poverty reduction. Though no data is available in Table 2, still poverty is acute in Afghanistan, where 80 per cent of the people live below the poverty line.

Table 2: Poverty Headcount Ratio at $1.90 a day (2011 ppp) (% of population) (1990-2018)

Country	1990	2000	2010	2018
Afghanistan	-	-	-	-
Bangladesh	44.2	34.8	19.6	14.8
Bhutan	-	17.6	2.2	1.5
India	45.9	-	21.2	-
Maldives	-	10.0	7.3	0.0
Nepal	-	49.9	15.0	-
Pakistan	58.9	28.6	8.3	3.9
Sri Lanka	8.7	8.3	2.4	0.8

Source: https://data.worldbank.org/country

Despite progress, South Asia still accounts for 40 per cent of the world's stunted children due to malnutrition. Women in the region suffer from anaemia due to lack of iron at still the world's highest rates (Fruman and Zhang 2020). The food security situation in contemporary South Asian countries is not satisfactory, which has deteriorated slightly between 2014 and 2018 (Table 2). For instance, *The State of Food Insecurity in the World 2015* report by the FAO et al. (2015) reveals that 'The highest burden of hunger in absolute terms is to be found in Southern Asia. Estimates for 2014–16 suggest that about 281 million people are undernourished in the region, marking only a slight reduction from the number in 1990–92, 291 million'. The World Bank notes that in 2015, half of the world's poor people were found in five countries, i.e., Bangladesh, India, Democratic Republic of Congo, Ethiopia, and Nigeria (World Bank 2018:29). In *The State of Food Security and Nutrition in the World 2019*, it is noted that 'Southern Asia is still the sub-region where the prevalence of undernourishment is highest [in Asia], at almost 15 percent' (FAO et al. 2019: xvii). FAO et al. (2019) note that the food security situation in South Asia between 2014 and 2018 has slightly deteriorated (Table 3).

Table 3: Number of People Experienced with Moderate or Severe Food Insecurity in South Asia (2014-2018)

Year	Number of severely food insecure people (in millions)	Number of moderately food insecure people (in millions)
2014	247.1	565.7
2015	225.4	561.3
2016	195.8	559.6
2017	204.2	525.8
2018	271.7	649.1

Source: FAO et al. 2019:18.

Table 3 demonstrates that both the number of severely and moderately food insecure people in South Asia has increased between 2014 and 2018 and that merits serious attention. The impact of COVID-19 will worsen the food security situation globally in general and South Asia in particular, which is explained in the following sections.

Implications of COVID-19 on Food Security

Food security was a significant challenge globally for more than 820 million people who suffered from hunger even before the novel coronavirus outbreak (Tiensin et al. 2020; Ewbank 2015). H.E. Tijjani

Muhammad Bande, President of the 74th Session of the United Nations General Assembly, notes that COVID-19 will 'hit the most vulnerable populations hardest. Before the spread of coronavirus, there were 2 billion people malnourished; and 700 million people lived below the poverty line' (Bande 2020). Notably, one in every nine persons did not have enough to eat. It is argued that 'Food security is one of the great issues of our time with all the available evidence suggesting that in most parts of the world, climate change is making the challenges of producing adequate food more difficult' (Connell and Lowitt 2020: v). South Asian countries are vulnerable to global warming and climate change. These countries are already facing severe consequences of climate change in agriculture production. COVID-19 global pandemic will make the situation worse as it is 'expected to be a key driver of acute food insecurity' (Barbiroglio 2020). Though no country or continent is immune to this, definitely the poor countries will be most vulnerable to food insecurity created by COVID-19 compared to the rich countries. In this regard, Cedric Habiyaremye, a research associate at Washington State University, rightly notes that 'Rural areas in those [sub-Saharan Africa] countries will be particularly vulnerable to food insecurity due to pandemic. Not only will the pandemic impact rural people's livelihoods (and therefore the demand for food), but it will also create barriers to accessing food, by restricting mobility and creating higher costs of doing business due to the tightening of credit' (cited in Barbiroglio 2020).

It is argued that '[d]uring the pandemic, the world's immediate focus has necessarily been on health and containing the spread of COVID-19. However, the economic shutdown poses a grave risk to food supply, production, and livelihoods' (Howard and Simmons 2020). According to the World Bank, 'as the coronavirus crisis unfolds, disruptions in domestic food supply chains and other shocks affecting food production and affordability are creating strong tensions and food security risks in many countries' (World Bank, April 23, 2020). Consequently, COVID-19 threatens global food security (Howard and Simmons 2020; Hamilton 2020). According to the United Nations World Food Programme, the number of people who face acute food insecurity will be doubled (pushing it to 265 million) by the end of 2020 due to the impacts of COVID-19 (WFP, April 21, 2020). WFP's Chief Economist, Arif Husain contends that

> COVID-19 is potentially catastrophic for millions who are already hanging by a thread. It is a hammer blow for millions more who can only eat if they earn a wage. Lockdowns and global economic recession have already decimated their nest eggs. It only takes one more shock—like COVID-19—to push them over the edge. We must collectively act now to mitigate the impact of this global catastrophe (WFP, April 21, 2020).

It also becomes essential to look at how COVID-19 impacts livelihoods and consequently, the food security of the people who work in informal sectors. According to the International Labour Organisation (2020:1) 'Among the most vulnerable in the labour market, almost 1.6 billion (nearly half of the global workforce) informal economy workers are significantly impacted by lockdown measures and/or working in the hardest-hit sectors'. Due to the COVID-19 global pandemic, the loss of livelihood or earnings will severely impact the food security of those people and their family members. One also needs to look at the impacts of COVID-19 on decline in remittances and increasing poverty as remittances contribute significantly in South Asian economies. Panu Poutvaara, an economist at the University of Munich and a member of the German Expert Council on Integration and Migration, contends that 'I do not expect widespread famine, but tens of millions more are likely to end up in severe poverty. Unfortunately, when the cut in remittances is combined with other shocks hitting poor countries, like the collapse of tourism and steep declines in exports, there is going to be a steep increase in global poverty' (cited in Lindsay 2020). He notes that 'it will last several years before pre-pandemic remittance levels are reached again' (quoted in Lindsay 2020). Jane Rabinowicz & Martin Settle write that 'Many food systems in the global South were already under stress before this crisis, due to climate change, migration, and political instability. The impacts of COVID-19 could take these already strained food systems beyond their breaking point' (Rabinowicz & Settle 2020). Therefore, COVID-19 will impact the food security of tens of thousands of people in the world in several ways, including disrupting food availability and reducing purchasing power capacity and thus impacting nutrition and stability.

COVID-19 and Food Security in South Asia

Poverty, hunger, malnutrition are some of the common features in South Asian countries despite progress made in poverty reduction in the last decades (Table 1). South Asia is already in a tense situation in terms of food security. The number of food insecure people is increasing in the region. In this context, the implications of the COVID-19 global pandemic might be devastating. Howard and Simmons (2020) contend that 'The loss of jobs and incomes is already reducing agriculture-related demand and threatening gains made on poverty and nutrition in South Asia...over the past decade'. In fact, one can understand the acute food insecurity in South Asia because of the COVID-19 global pandemic through looking at some selected headlines that appeared in the media (Table 4).

Table 4: Some Selected Headlines of Food Insecurity in South Asia due to COVID-19

Headlines	Country	Source & date
Kerala: Workers' protest over lack of food supply enters Day 2	India	*The Indian Express*, March 31, 2020
Hungry amid shutdown, Narayanganj's poor take protest to streets	Bangladesh	*The Business Standard*, April 8, 2020.
Queues from 6 am for lunch in Delhi as lockdown hits the poorest	India	*NDTV*, April 13, 2020
Khulna's workless, hungry people take protest to street	Bangladesh	*The Business Standard*, April 14, 2020.
Coronavirus: Hungry people demonstrate for food in Jashore	Bangladesh	*UNB News*, April 15, 2020
Long queues in the sun for a meal, yet hundreds go hungry in Chandigarh	India	*Hindustan Times*, April 15, 2020
COVID-19: Thousands take to streets demanding relief, food	Bangladesh	*Dhaka Tribune*, April 16, 2020
Hunger grows in Mumbai: Working poor now queuing up for free food	India	*The Indian Express*, April 16, 2020
People go on protests for relief in dists	Bangladesh	*New Age*, April 17, 2020
Hundreds protest for food in Narayanganj	Bangladesh	*Dhaka Tribune*, April 18, 2020
Watch: In Delhi, hungry people join a 2-km-long food queue in peak afternoon sun	India	Scroll.in, April 18, 2020

(Contd.)

Headlines	Country	Source & date
Food looted in Chattogram: Protests for relief go on in districts	Bangladesh	*New Age*, April 19, 2020
Coronavirus: Unemployed locals seeking food aid demonstrate in Jessore	Bangladesh	*Dhaka Tribune*, April 22, 2020.
A thousand protest demanding food aid	Bangladesh	*The Daily Star*, April 28, 2020
Khulna residents and transportation workers protest for food relief	Bangladesh	*The Business Standard*, May 6, 2020
Transport workers in hardship, protest for food aid at Gabtoli	Bangladesh	*The New Nation*, May 6, 2020
Coronavirus: Six killed in clashes at Afghanistan food aid protest	Afghanistan	*BBC News*, May 9, 2020
Video shows migrants fighting over packet of food at Bihar train station	India	*NDTV*, May 14, 2020
COVID-19 lockdown: Migrants protest near Madhya Pradesh-Maharashtra border over food, transport	India	Scroll.in, May 15, 2020

Table 4 demonstrates that there were protests, fights, clashes, looting for food in South Asian countries particularly in Bangladesh and India. In fact, the two kilometre-long queue for free meal distribution demonstrates the acute food insecurity in South Asia due to the COVID-19 global pandemic. This chapter discusses in detail the impacts of the COVID-19 global pandemic in food security in South Asia in the following sub-sections.

Food Availability

One needs to look at the first dimension of food security, i.e., availability of food supply in the markets of South Asia. Thus, it becomes pertinent to look at how does the novel coronavirus impact food supply availability in South Asia. One can argue that food supply availability will be affected in South Asia through supply chain shock. Lockdown measures and business closures in the South Asian region created impediments in the movement of commodities to consumers. Thus, the supply chain shock due to the transportation, physical and economic restrictions have already created unemployment problems in the region. The collapse of global markets due to COVID-19 has multiplied the vulnerability of the supply chain (especially ready-made garments) workers in South Asia substantially in the domain of food security. In addition, it is noted that 'a range of informal and small and medium scale businesses constitute the great majority of the food system—providing production, processing, marketing, and food services, including street food vendors and restaurants. Their inability to operate will affect food access throughout major population centres' (Howard and Simmons 2020). In this regard, the World Food Programme notes that 'movement restrictions necessary to contain the spread of the virus will disrupt the transport and processing of food and other critical goods, increasing delivery times and reducing the availability of even the most basic food items'. Julie Howard and Emmy Simmons, Senior Adviser at Global Food Security Programme, write that 'Delays in deliveries of essential foods and agricultural inputs will affect food supplies for many months to come' (Howard and Simmons 2020).

Agriculture is labour-intensive in South Asia. Thus, labour shortages due to the weeks-long lockdown measures impact agriculture production, rice, wheat, maize harvesting. Notably, April-May is the peak season for rice harvesting in many parts of South Asia. In Bangladesh, due to weeks-long lockdown, migrant labourers are not able to travel, which created a labour shortage for harvesting. The picture is similar in the case of India (Tewary 2020). In Pakistan, around 70 per cent of small-scale farmers rely on migratory farm labourers who have been unable to travel, according to the *Anadolu Agency*. Ahmad Ali, a farmer from Pakistan's north-eastern Punjab province, points out that 'There is an acute shortage of labour here. I am completely clueless what to do' (*Anadolu Agency*, April 10, 2020). Like Ali, there are tens of thousands of farmers who are not getting the required labour force for rice, wheat, maize harvesting. Many labourers are scared of getting infected with coronavirus which is also contributing to the labour shortages.

The lockdown crisis has impacted millions of farmers in the region negatively as their agro products go unsold or are poorly paid for. For instance, the *Financial Express* (April 21, 2020) in its editorial, writes that 'farmers in some major vegetable growing districts including Rajshahi,

Rangpur, Dinajpur, Bogura, Manikganj, Cumilla, Narsingdi, Jashore, Khulna and Chattogram could not even get one fourth of their production costs by selling their crops in the market'. Thus, small-scale farmers are severely affected in Bangladesh due to supply chain shock (*Daily Ittefaq*, April 20, 2020). Additionally, dairy farmers in Bangladesh were not able to sell milk as the sweets-producer factories, and local hotels had been closed down. The picture in other South Asian countries is similar. For instance, after interviewing 150 small farmers in Assam, it is reported that they have grown vegetables that remain unsold amid lockdown. Each farmer would lose about US$ 263 (Rs. 20,000), which severely affects them and their families (Mander and Azad 2020). Aakash Patel, a farmer from Sagar district in central Madhya Pradesh state, told *Anadolu Agency* that 'We cannot sell those [vegetables] due to the lockdown. No means of transport is available to take them to wholesale markets. We pluck cabbages, cauliflowers, and other vegetables but are forced to feed them to the cattle' (*Anadolu Agency*, April 10, 2020). Zahid Bhurgari, a farmer from Pakistan's southern Mirpur Khas district, contends that 'On the one hand the prices of vegetables have decreased due to closure of hotels, restaurants, and banquets; on the other, the absence of transport due to lockdown is acting as a double whammy. Even the transport available is costing us three times the actual cost. We are left with no other option, but to leave the crops to rot in the fields' (*Anadolu Agency*, April 10, 2020). This will impact both the supply chain and the purchasing capacity of small-scale farmers as their agro produce remains unsold.

In the short term, the availability of food in the market is also impacted by panic-buying by consumers. Amid the COVID-19 crisis, it is reported that in many places, some affluent consumers bought excessive amounts of food. This panic-buying by some (rich) consumers created a crisis of food for other customers. It is rightly noted that 'In some places, nutritious food is becoming scarce. Among other concerns, food is being hoarded, leaving little on shelves for consumers' (Tiensin et al. 2020). As a result of such crisis, food prices get higher, which made food unaffordable for many middle-income and lower-income poor people. This also increases the vulnerability to coronavirus as malnourished individuals with compromised immunity are more at risk and susceptible to its spread (Global Alliance for Improved Nutrition 2020).

Availability of food will also be affected by the export ban and border closures due to the COVID-19 global pandemic. Many countries banned exports, including rice, wheat, and eggs, in order to guarantee food security for their own countries. According to one European rice trader, 'If Vietnam maintains the export ban we will suddenly have about 10-15 per cent less available supply in the world market in the near term. Africa especially could face disruption from this' (Thukral and Dahan 2020). Against the food export ban, Amina Mohamed writes that 'the proliferation of such measures could negatively affect the food security of countries that depend on international trade for the bulk of their needs—including many of Africa's least-developed economies' (Mohamed 2020). It is likely that South Asian countries will also be affected due to the export ban and border closures by many considering the interconnected nature of the global market.

Accessibility of Food
Sonu Singh (30) was working as a garment worker in Delhi since 1999 who never begged for food. Singh lost his job and the roof over his head due to the lockdown measures. Consequently, COVID-19 made him beg for food from door to doors in Jangpura, Delhi. Though he managed some food for himself, he could not ensure food for his wife and one-year-old daughter who live at home in Etah district, Uttarakhand (Baruah 2020). This is how the novel coronavirus impacts the accessibility of food of the tens of thousands of poor, marginal people in South Asia.

COVID-19 impacts the accessibility of food through hurting the purchasing capacity. In fact, the purchasing capacity of the people in South Asia depends on the sustainability of their jobs/earning sources. The implications of COVID-19 on food security are particularly severe for South Asian countries where almost half of the world's hungry people reside. One needs to look at the implications of COVID-19 on the rising unemployment and under-employment in South Asia. Lockdown measures and business closures created tens of thousands of people unemployed in South Asia who mostly work in the informal sector. For instance, according to the Biruni Institute, a local economic think-tank, six million people have already lost their jobs in Afghanistan due to the COVID-19 global pandemic (Pikulicka-Wilczewska 2020). Notably, 80 per cent of people live below the poverty line in Afghanistan. Thus, food security of tens of thousands of Afghans becomes a grave concern due to the pandemic. Additionally, the prices of food in Afghanistan have increased, which goes beyond the purchasing capacity of many. Many people are forced to beg in the streets due to the acute food insecurity brought by coronavirus. Thus, in Afghanistan, many believe that if coronavirus does not, poverty will kill them (Pikulicka-Wilczewska 2020). Inzar Gul Safi, an internally displaced person, points out that, 'We have no oil, no bread, and so far no coronavirus. The government recommends that we should take Vitamin C, eat oranges, to protect ourselves. However, how can we afford it?' (cited in Pikulicka-Wilczewska 2020).

The Daily Star reports that more than 10 million people who work in the informal sector have lost their livelihoods in Bangladesh due to the coronavirus outbreak (Parvez 2020). To contain the coronavirus spread, factories have been closed down in South Asian countries which have brought enormous challenges for the factory workers. Daily wage earners who work in informal economies are mostly in danger due to the impacts of the COVID-19 global pandemic. In addition, global buyers have cancelled orders, which impacted local garment owners. It is seen that many garment workers protested in Bangladesh in April and May 2020 to receive their salaries. As factories have been shut down, tens of thousands of factory workers have no money to buy food.

In the case of India, according to a survey by CMIE, 44 per cent households reported a loss of income, up from around 10 per cent in early March (cited in Rao 2020). In another telephonic survey by the National Council of Applied Economic Research in Delhi, it was found that 84 per cent of respondents reported loss of income, and nearly 30 per cent experienced shortages of food, fuel, and medicines (cited in Rao 2020). According to a survey by the Ministry of Health, India, 44 per cent people remain starved in India due to lockdown (*Ananda Bazar Patrika*, April 28, 2020).

It is also essential to look at how COVID-19 impacts remittances. The World Bank forecasts that there will be a 20 per cent decline in global remittances in 2020 due to the economic recession caused by COVID-19 (World Bank, April 22, 2020). Many South Asian households rely on remittances to meet their basic necessities. In 2018, Afghanistan received US$ 804 million, Bangladesh received US$ 15,562 million, Bhutan received US$ 58 million, India received US$ 78,790 million, Maldives received US$ 4 million, Nepal received US$ 8,294 million, Pakistan received US$ 21,194 million, and Sri Lanka received US$ 7,043 million as remittances (https://data.worldbank.org/country). In 2019, South Asia received remittances of US$ 140 billion. It is projected that South Asia will lose 22.1 per cent (US$ 109 billion) of remittances in 2020 due to COVID-19 (World Bank, April 22, 2020). Thus, when South Asian expatriates lose jobs in the Middle East or Gulf countries due to lockdown measures and factory, business closures, it will severely impact the food and nutrition security of many households in the home countries. It is reported that many South Asian migrants are forced to leave Middle Eastern countries due to allegations of infection even without testing all (Budhathoki 2020).

One can also argue that movement restrictions of labour can lead to shortages of food in the market, which will impact prices. If food prices increase, accessibility also becomes challenging for the poor and marginal. Thus, lockdown measures and factory closures created acute food insecurity for workers and their family members. Additionally, social safety net programmes are weak in the South Asian region. There is also a lack of transparency in distributing government relief. One also needs to understand the COVID-19 impacts on the utilisation and nutrition aspects of food security.

One also needs to look at the impacts of rising food prices on the accessibility of food. In fact, rising food prices impact the poor severely. The 2008 global economic recession that resulted in increased food prices which even resulted in riots in some parts of the world demonstrated the importance of sustainable food security. Again, after the outbreak of novel coronavirus in South Asia, the prices of essential foods have increased. For instance, due to border and business closures to curb the spread of COVID-19, food prices increased substantially in South Asian countries. In mid-March, when the Afghanistan-Pakistan border was closed to contain the spread of COVID-19, food prices in Afghanistan jumped by up to 30 per cent overnight (Amani 2020).

Nutrition Access and Food Utilisation

Adequate nutrition access becomes vital for a child's brain development and physical, mental, and cognitive development. Lack of nutrition leads to stunting and underweight in children. Malnutrition becomes a prime driver for poor health outcomes, i.e., reduced productivity. According to FAO (2018: 4), 'Nutritional deficits in the first 1,000 days of life imply long-term developmental problems'. COVID-19 impedes nutrition access of the people in South Asia. While people are concerned about two meals a day, access to nutrition becomes a luxury for many people in South Asia. As noted earlier, many poor and marginal people are suffering from acute hunger during lockdown days; access to nutritious foods becomes a dream. Even for tens of thousands of children in South Asia, access to one egg or a piece of fish in the meal becomes very challenging. For instance, Miya Gul, who has six children, contends that 'We buy one potato for 10 Afghani [$ 0.13]. People who have money can buy a kilo. And we can afford only one per day' (cited in Pikulicka-Wilczewska 2020). Gul's family is facing starvation as 'coronavirus lockdown has wiped out jobs' (Pikulicka-Wilczewska 2020). Like Gul, there are many South Asians who are not able to buy food for their family members. For them, access to nutritious food becomes a real challenge. One can also argue that children in South Asia will be the worst hit due to the COVID-19 global pandemic in the context of access to nutrition. As many earning members would lose their sources of income due to the pandemic, children from those poor families would be forced into child labour which would affect their nutrition access severely.

Access to clean water and proper sanitation services also becomes vital in the domain of food security. It is noted that 'Every day, more than two billion people around the world are forced to drink contaminated water. Diarrhoea caused by contaminated water and poor sanitation kills a child under five years old every two minutes' (Barlow 2020). COVID-19 'puts the human right to water, front and centre' (Barlow 2020). In the pre-pandemic time, food utilisation was not satisfactory for many South Asian countries (Table 3). The COVID-19 global pandemic impacts food utilisation severely as the livelihood security of many is threatened in South Asia.

Table 3: Access to Basic Drinking Water and Sanitation Services in South Asian Countries in 2017

Country	Access to basic drinking water services	Access to basic sanitation services
Afghanistan	67.1	43.4
Bangladesh	97	48.2
Bhutan	97.2	69.3
India	92.7	59.5
Maldives	99.3	99.4
Nepal	88.8	62.1
Pakistan	91.5	59.9
Sri Lanka	89.4	95.8

Source: FAOSTAT, http://www.fao.org/faostat/en/#country

What is to be Done

Prioritising Agriculture

To address the consequences in COVID-19 in the food production system, agriculture needs to be prioritised in the national budget. Swaminathan and Rao (2020) write that 'farmers are confronted at the moment with labour shortages, many of the inputs, including seeds, are expensive or unavailable, marketing arrangements including supply chains are not fully functional, pricing is not remunerative, and public procurement is also not adequate'. Consequently, sufficient stimulus packages, agriculture subsidies, seeds distribution, machinery, i.e., tractors need to be distributed among the farmers. They can be given loans with lower or without interest rates. South Asia is primarily an agriculture-based economy. Thus, if farmers are not protected, both the short term and long term food security of the people in the region will be threatened. *The Financial Express* (April 21, 2020) in its editorial writes that 'it is of utmost importance that farmers get direct cash subsidy to continue with their role of feeding the nation with vitamin-enriched victuals'. Thus, it is strongly suggested that there is no alternative to increase investments in agriculture to overcome future food insecurity in South Asia.

Stabilising Food System and Keeping Trade Open

Many argue that strong nationalism, protectionist trade policy, strong borders, restricted movements of goods and people due to the COVID-19 global pandemic will negatively impact the global food system. Thus, in both short and long term, it becomes important to stabilise the food system and keep trade open locally, regionally and globally. From farmers to shopkeepers and supermarket agents, all are critical to keeping the food system moving. Thus, in the COVID-19 and post COVID-19 global pandemic situations, it becomes crucial to ensure the food security and well-being of these people. Tiensin et al. (2020) write in *Project Syndicate* that 'Like medical care, food must be allowed to cross borders freely. Food producers must ensure that healthy, nutritious foods are available and not wasted'. It is also important to avoid panic buying and wasting of food by consumers.

Many countries have restricted exporting food items. Vietnam, the third-largest rice exporter, has suspended rice export contracts temporarily. Kazakhstan, one of the most significant sources of wheat flour, has banned exporting it along with buckwheat and vegetables, i.e., onions, carrots, and potatoes (Harvey 2020). In this regard, H.E. Tijjani Muhammad Bande, President of the 74th Session of the United Nations General Assembly argues that 'Trade restrictions can trigger shortages and inflate the prices of food items abruptly' (Bande 2020). Similarly, Maximo Torero, chief economist of the UN Food and Agriculture Organisation, warns that 'Trade barriers will create extreme volatility. [They] will make the situation worse. That's what we observe in food crises' (Harvey 2020). Thus, instead of following a protectionist policy, states of the world need to deepen cooperation on trade. In fact, trade can help to prevent food disaster in the making.

Strengthening Economy
Sustainable economic growth is crucial for food security in South Asia. But it is worrying that many are arguing for the protectionist policy after the outbreak of coronavirus. But for the long term solutions of food insecurity, it becomes essential to have a strong economy in the South Asian countries. In fact, free trade is important. It becomes worthy to note that Sèna Kimm Gnangnon studies the impact of multilateral trade liberalisation on the economic growth rate by using a dataset comprising 150 countries over the period between 1995 and 2015. Gnangnon (2018) finds that there is a 'strong positive impact' of trade liberation on the economic growth of the countries. Many countries around the world, including the USA, have lifted themselves out of poverty due to their embracing the free market economy. Gary Hufbauer (2008) writes that 'In fact, free trade has increased American household income by lowering costs of products, increasing wages and making more-efficient American companies'.

Strengthening Social Safety Net Programmes
It is argued that '[t]he virus has resulted in mass unemployment and further threatens millions of jobs. Given the intrinsic link between poverty and food security, we must prioritise social protection measures which will safeguard the most vulnerable, including those working in the informal economy; and women who are also disproportionately affected' (Bande 2020). It is important to bring transparency in social safety programmes. Since South Asian states have limited resources, regional and international institutions, i.e., SAARC, BIMSTEC, ASEAN, World Bank, IMF, AIIB, WFP need to come forward to strengthen social safety net programmes in South Asia based on transparency and win-win situations.

Promoting Regional Cooperation
Politics in South Asia contributes to food insecurity for many. In fact,

absence of regional cooperation on agriculture, water and other areas including the regional food bank work as major impediments to ensure food security in South Asia to a large extent. Sneyed et al (2015) observes that food security is political. From the theorisation of the term 'food security,' its implementation is quite political. Against the backdrop of the export ban of major agriculture producers, there is no alternative to deepen cooperation among South Asian countries in terms of seeds distribution, research cooperation, technology sharing, economic cooperation. Additionally, South Asian countries need to remove tariffs and non-tariff barriers and simplify Customs clearance procedures for imports of agricultural products, essential drugs and equipment. Specifically, the negative list of agro-products needs to be addressed. Thus, South Asian countries also need to concentrate on operationalising the (South Asian Free Trade Arrangement) and other relevant SAARC agencies. Intra-trade among the countries of the region is at minimal level which also merits urgent attention. In the post-COVID-19 world, South Asian leaders, academics, civil society organisations, epistemic communities need to deepen cooperation at the regional level to face future food insecurity arising from COVID-19. It becomes vital to keep people in the centre of South Asian politics. One can argue that SAARC food bank needs to be functional to face any future pandemic or shocks. In addition, deepening connectivity can be another important area of food security cooperation in the region, since poor connectivity leads to increased transportation costs, which increase the price of food grains. This ultimately leads to food insecurity. Water is a crucial element required for food production. But unfortunately, water governance in the region is poor. And hence, the region should concentrate on proper water governance. One can also add that South Asia needs a common stance on WTO negotiations regarding agriculture subsidies.

Conclusion

The chapter found that the COVID-19 global pandemic has devastating impacts on the food security of South Asian people especially for the poor and marginalised. In the case of making policies on food security in South Asia during the pandemic and post-pandemic period, the nutrition and utilisation aspects need to be emphasised which often goes overlooked. The rise of strong/extreme nationalism, and thus a protectionist trade policy, travel restrictions, suspended flight operations, border closures and labour shortages disrupt local, regional, and global food supply chains. It impacts food security drastically which requires cooperation from all: both from states and non-state actors. The bottom line is that in the post-COVID-19 world, South Asian states need to concentrate on ensuring food and nutrition security by prioritising agriculture in the national budget and deepening food security cooperation regionally.

REFERENCES

Amani, W. (2020, April 17). A Hunger Crisis Beckons as Afghans Reel From the Impact of COVID-19. *The Diplomat*. Retrieved from https://thediplomat.com/2020/04/a-hunger-crisis-beckons-as-afghans-reel-from-the-impact-of-COVID-19/

Ananda Bazar Patrika (2020, April 28). India lockdown: Half of the mass remains starved [In Bangla]. Retrieved from https://www.anandabazar.com/national/india-lockdown-half-of-the-mass-remains-starved-due-to-food-crisis-1.1142654

Anadolu Agency (2020, April 10). COVID-19 lockdown sparks harvest crises in Pakistan, India: In absence of labour, transport, fear of pandemic, farmers staring at disaster, as nations head for possible food shortage. Retrieved from https://www.aa.com.tr/en/asia-pacific/COVID-19-lockdown-sparks-harvest-crises-in-pakistan-india/1799536

Bande, T. M. (2020, April 17). The impact of COVID-19 on global food security and nutrition: Preventing a health crisis from becoming a food crisis. President of the 74th Session, United Nations General Assembly. Retrieved from https://www.un.org/pga/74/2020/04/17/the-impact-of-COVID-19-on-global-food-security-and-nutrition-preventing-a-health-crisis-from-becoming-a-food-crisis/

Barbiroglio, E. (2020, April 23). COVID-19 is expected to be a key driver of acute food insecurity. *Forbes*. Retrieved from https://www.forbes.com/sites/emanuelabarbiroglio/2020/04/23/COVID-19-is-expected-to-be-a-key-driver-of-acute-food-insecurity/#a1647f478ef7

Baruah, S. (2020, April 29). Delhi: Once a jeans factory worker, man goes door to door in Jangpura in search of food. *The Indian Express*. Retrieved from https://indianexpress.com/article/cities/delhi/delhi-once-a-jeans-factory-worker-man-goes-door-to-door-in-jangpura-in-search-of-food-6383921/

Barlow, M. (2020, April 22). COVID-19 puts the human right to water front and centre. *National Observer*. Retrieved from https://www.nationalobserver.com/2020/04/22/opinion/COVID-19-puts-human-right-water-front-and-centre

Budhathoki, A. (2020, April 24). Middle East autocrats target South Asian workers. *The Business Standard*. Retrieved from https://tbsnews.net/coronavirus-chronicle/middle-east-autocrats-target-south-asian-workers-73429

Burgess, J. P. (2012). Introduction. In J. P. Burgess (Ed.), *The Routledge Handbook of New Security Studies*, (pp.1-4). Abingdon, Oxon: Routledge.

Connell, J. and Lowitt, K. (2020). Preface. In J. Connell and K. Lowitt (Eds.), *Food Security in Small Island States*. (pp.v-vi), Gateway East, Singapore: Springer Nature.

Daily Ittefaq (2020, April 20). Vegetable farmers are in danger [In Bangla]. Retrieved from https://www.ittefaq.com.bd/wholecountry/145929/%E0%A7% A8% E0% A7%A8-%E0%A6%AC%E0%A6%B8%E0%A7%8D%E0%A6%A4% E0% A6%BE-%E0%A6%AC%E0%A7%87%E0%A6%97%E0%A7%81%E0%A6%A8-%E0%A7%AB%E0%A7%A6%E0%A7%A6-%E0% A6%9 F% E0% A6% BE% E0% A6%95% E0%A6%BE%E0%A7%9F-%E0%A6%AA%E0%A7%8D%E0%A6% B0% E0%A6%A4%E0%A6%BF-%E0%A6%AA%E0%A6%BF%E0%A6%B8-%E0%A6%B2%E0%A6%BE%E0%A6%89-%E0% A6% A4% E0% A6% BF% E0% A6%A8-%E0%A6%9F%E0%A6%BE%E0%A6%95%E0%A6%BE%E0%A7%9F-%E0%A6%AC%E0%A6%BF%E0%A6%95%E0%A7%8D%E0%A6%B0%E0%A6%BF

Ewbank, R. (2015, July 29). Just growing more food won't help to feed the world. *The Guardian*, 29 July. Retrieved from http://www.theguardian.com/global-development/2015/jul/29/growing-more-food-wont-help-feed-world-agriculture-climate-resilient

FAO (2010). *The State of Food Insecurity in the World 2010*. Rome, FAO.

FAO, IFAD and WFP. (2015). *The State of Food Insecurity in the World 2015. Meeting the 2015 international hunger targets: taking stock of uneven progress*. Rome: FAO.

FAO (2018). *State of Food and Agriculture in Asia and the Pacific Region, including Future Prospects and Emerging Issues*. FAO regional conference for Asia and the Pacific. Thirty-fourth Session, Nadi, Fiji, 9–13 April.

FAO, IFAD, UNICEF, WFP and WHO. (2019). *The state of food security and nutrition in the world 2019. Safeguarding against economic slowdowns and downturns*. Rome, FAO. Licence: CC BY-NC-SA 3.0 IGO.

Financial Times (2020, April 21). Warnings of unrest mount as coronavirus hits food availability. Retrieved from https://www.ft.com/content/443b74f7-e9f2-412f-b9d6-241168cc1710

Fruman, C. & Zhang, Y. (2020, May 5). Ensuring food security and nutrition in South Asia during COVID-19. World Bank Blogs. Retrieved from https://blogs.worldbank.org/endpovertyinsouthasia/ensuring-food-security-and-nutrition-south-asia-during-COVID-19

George, P. S. (1994). Food security in South Asia: Performance and prospects. *Economic and Political Weekly*, 29(18): 1092-1094.

Global Alliance for Improved Nutrition (2020, March 23). The COVID-19 crisis and food systems: addressing threats, creating opportunities. Retrieved from https://www.gainhealth.org/media/news/COVID-19-crisis-and-food-systems-addressing-threats-creating-opportunities

Gnangnon, S. K. (2018). Multilateral trade liberalization and economic growth. *Journal of Economic Integration*. 33 (2), 1261-1301.

Hamilton, P. C. (2020, April 14). COVID-19 and food security in vulnerable countries. United Nations Conference on Trade and Development. Retrieved from https://unctad.org/en/pages/newsdetails.aspx?OriginalVersionID=2331

Harvey, F. (2020, March 26). Coronavirus measures could cause global food shortage, UN warns. *The Guardian*. Retrieved from https://www.theguardian.com/global-development/2020/mar/26/coronavirus-measures-could-cause-global-

food-shortage-un-warns
Howard, J. and Simmons, E. (2020, April 22). COVID-19 threatens global food security: What should the United States do? Centre for Strategic and International Studies. Retrieved from https://www.csis.org/analysis/COVID-19-threatens-global-food-security-what-should-united-states-do
Hufbauer, G. (2008). Free trade. *The National Interest*, 95, 15-18.
International Labour Organization (2020, April 29). *ILO Monitor*: COVID-19 and the world of work. Third edition.
Lindsay, F. (2020, April 22). World Bank: Global Remittances Set To Decline Sharply As A Result of Coronavirus. *Forbes*. Retrieved from https://www.forbes.com/sites/freylindsay/2020/04/22/world-bank-global-remittances-set-to-decline-sharply-as-a-result-of-coronavirus/#3fad851a60ab
Mander, H. and Azad, A. K. (2020, April 13). 'I cannot eat or sleep': In Assam, farmers grow anxious as vegetables go unsold amid lockdown. *Scroll.in*. Retrieved from https://scroll.in/article/958955/i-cannot-eat-or-sleep-in-assam-farmers-grown-anxious-as-vegetables-go-unsold-amid-lockdown
Maxwell, S. (1996). Food security: A post-modern perspective. *Food Policy* 21(2), 155–70.
McLachlan, M.& Hamann, R. (2011). Theme issue on food security. *Development Southern Africa*, 28(4), 429-430, DOI: 10.1080/0376835X.2011.605558
Mohamed, A. (2020, April 24). Protectionism Is No Cure for Pandemics. Project Syndicate. Retrieved from https://www.project-syndicate.org/commentary/protectionism-will-prolong-the-covid19-pandemic-by-amina-mohamed-2020-04
Nicholson, L. (2020, April 10). Sign of the times: Mile-long line of cars outside California grocery giveaway. Reuters. Retrieved from https://www.reuters.com/article/us-health-coronavirus-usa-food/sign-of-the-times-mile-long-line-of-cars-outside-california-grocery-giveaway-idUSKCN21R3N3
Parvez, S. (2020, May 1). More than a crore with no job and hope. *The Daily Star*. Retrieved from https://www.thedailystar.net/business/news/more-crore-no-job-and-hope-1898554
Pikulicka-Wilczewska, A. (2020, May 8). Afghans face dire condition in Ramadan amid coronavirus lockdown. *Al Jazeera*. Retrieved from https://www.aljazeera.com/news/2020/04/afghans-face-dire-condition-ramadan-coronavirus-lockdown-200430114049678.html
Pinstrup-Andersen, P. (2009). Food security: definition and measurement. *Food Security*, (1), 5–7. DOI 10.1007/s12571-008-0002-y
Rabinowicz, J. & Settle, M. (2020, April 22). COVID-19 is creating a food crisis and Canada needs to respond. *National Observer*. Retrieved from https://www.nationalobserver.com/2020/04/22/opinion/COVID-19-creating-food-crisis-and-canada-needs-respond
Rao, K. (2020, April 27). Protecting the poor from becoming poorer. *The Hindu*. Retrieved from https://www.thehindu.com/opinion/op-ed/protecting-the-poor-from-becoming-poorer/article31439214.ece
Shepherd, B. (2012). Thinking critically about food security. *Security Dialogue*, 43(3), 195–212.
Sneyd, A., Legwegoh, A. F. & Sneyd, L. Q. (2015). Food politics: perspectives on food security in Central Africa, *Journal of Contemporary African Studies*, 33(1), 141-161.
Swaminathan, M. S. & Rao, N. (2020, May 2). It's about food, nutrition and livelihood

security. *The Hindu*. Retrieved from https://www.thehindu.com/opinion/lead/its-about-food-nutrition-and-livelihood-security/article31484674.ece

Tewary, A. (2020, April 4). Bihar farmers facing serious labour crunch due to lockdown. *The Hindu*. Retrieved from https://www.thehindu.com/news/national/other-states/bihar-farmers-facing-serious-labour-crunch-due-to-lockdown/article31255288.ece

The Financial Express Editorial (2020, April 21). Helping out vegetable farmers. Retrieved from https://thefinancialexpress.com.bd/editorial/helping-out-vegetable-farmers-1587484077

The Guardian (2020, May 9). 'Hundreds queue for food parcels in wealthy Geneva. Retrieved from https://www.theguardian.com/world/2020/may/09/food-parcels-handed-out-to-workers-in-geneva-impacted-by-COVID-19

Thukral, N. and Dahan, M. E. (2020, March 26). Food security concerns stoked as exporters curb sales, importers buy more. *Reuters*. Retrieved from https://www.reuters.com/article/us-health-coronavirus-food-security/food-security-concerns-stoked-as-exporters-curb-sales-importers-buy-more-idUSKBN21D0YV

Tiensin, T., Kalibata, A. &, Cole, M. (2020, April 1). Ensuring Food Security in the Era of COVID-19. Project Syndicate. Retrieved from https://www.project-syndicate.org/commentary/covid19-threatens-to-unleash-global-food-insecurity-by-thanawat-tiensin-et-al-2020-03

Timmer, C. Peter (2015). *Food security and scarcity: Why ending hunger is so hard*, Philadelphia, Pennsylvania: University of Pennsylvania Press.

WFP (2020, April 21). COVID-19 will double number of people facing food crises unless swift action is taken. Retrieved from https://www.wfp.org/news/COVID-19-will-double-number-people-facing-food-crises-unless-swift-action-taken

Wiggings, S. & Slater, R. (2012). Food security. In J. P. Burgess (Ed.), *The Routledge Handbook of new Security Studies*, (pp.132-143). Abingdon, Oxon: Routledge.

World Bank (2018). *Poverty and shared prosperity 2018: Piecing together the poverty puzzle*. Washington, DC: World Bank. License: Creative Commons Attribution CC BY 3.0 IGO

World Bank (2020, April 22). World Bank predicts sharpest decline of remittances in recent history. Retrieved from https://www.worldbank.org/en/news/press-release/2020/04/22/world-bank-predicts-sharpest-decline-of-remittances-in-recent-history

World Bank (2020, April 23). Food security and COVID-19. Retrieved from https://www.worldbank.org/en/topic/agriculture/brief/food-security-and-COVID-19

Worldometers (n.d.). Southern Asia Population. Retrieved from https://www.worldometers.info/world-population/southern-asia-population/

Yaro, J. A. 2004. Theorizing food insecurity: building a livelihood vulnerability framework for researching food insecurity. *NorskGeografiskTidsskrift–Norwegian Journal of Geography, 58*, 23–37.

Websites

World Bank country profile, https://data.worldbank.org/country

FAOSTAT, http://www.fao.org/faostat/en/#country

4

Economic Security in South Asia

ABSTRACT

South Asia faces several challenges of economic security, which include poverty, inequality, and injustice, as seen in the everyday life of millions of people. Unemployment, low wages, discrimination, corruption, and rent-seeking continuously loom large in the living conditions of more than ninety-five per cent of the people. This chapter investigates the linkage between COVID-19 crisis and economic security in South Asia. How does COVID-19 influence economic security in South Asia? What might be the possible policy responses to address the implications of COVID-19 on South Asian economic security both in the short and long terms? This chapter addresses these questions based on the desk review. It argues that South Asia has been severely affected due to the impact of COVID-19 on different dimensions of the economy—trade, investment, aid and technology. It demonstrates that without due attention to the sources of economic insecurity in South Asia, no sustainable progress will be achieved.

Keywords: *COVID-19, Economic Security, South Asia, Global Economy and Recession.*

Introduction

The Japan Times ran a story on 29 April 2020 with the headline, 'Should I buy a mask or food? South Asia's poor face stark choice'. The story goes, 'Buy a mask and let his family go hungry, or buy food and go out into the crowded city without one—that is the stark choice facing Hayatullah Khan, an Afghan labourer whose daily earnings have fallen below $1.50 during the coronavirus pandemic' (Aneez and Saif 2020). This underlines the fact of the criticality of economic security in South Asia. Economic security is a major issue in South Asia in the context of socio-economic conditions as evolved over the decades. The continuing presence of massive poverty despite improvement and progress in the recent years makes the issue a top priority for the nations in South Asia. Since the end of the Cold War, economic security came to the centre-stage of domestic and international domains of policy making. In the process of broadening and deepening of security pioneered by Barry Buzan, economic issues and concerns had been considered from a security perspective (1987, 1991, 1997). South Asia as a region suffers from an array of intra-state and inter-state conflicts and challenges rooted in economic conditions. As post-colonial societies, South Asian economic conditions did not witness the emancipation that the leaders and activists imagined during their freedom struggle in the subcontinent. Hence, economic security remains a critical issue in the region.

The COVID-19 pandemic has created a new reality for South Asia. The Spanish flu of 1918 reportedly killed over 20 million people in South Asia, while the number of total deaths was reported about 50 million globally (Chhibber 2020). It is surprising that South Asia has fewer infections and deaths compared with North America and Western Europe. The unprecedented spread of the COVID-19 pandemic in the world covering 213 countries and regions has posed a great challenge to the entire humanity, perhaps not much in terms of the number of deaths, but in terms of the colossal impact on the highly integrated global economy. As far as the impact of the COVID-19 pandemic is concerned, analysts argue that it is going to be profound in all aspects of state and economy. From an economic perspective, Selim Raihan succinctly captures it:

> The global economy is facing "a double crisis" of an unmatched magnitude—the danger to public health due to the pandemic, and a growing risk of global economic recession. It is now commonly agreed that COVID-19's blow to the global economy will be stronger and sharper than the global financial crisis of 2008 and even the Great

Depression in the 1930s. To be precise, each part of the aggregate demand—consumption, investment, and exports—is being badly affected in most of the countries. Also, domestic, regional and global supply chains are severely disrupted, and it may take a long time to get back to the normal state (Raihan 2020).

South Asia has integrated its economy with the global economic system for the last three decades due to globalisation and interdependence. Trade, investment and technology as the engines of economic growth in South Asia are particularly connected with the global economy. Liberalisation of South Asian economies has opened up private sectors and eventually has established a dominance of the market economy in all countries in the region. Apparently, South Asia has benefitted from this openness and liberalisation in its macroeconomic dimension. The miraculous economic progress in the region over the last decade is attributed to South Asia's integration with the global economy based on the process of globalisation. At the same time, South Asia as a region is marked by poverty, inequality, corruption and injustice. It creates a puzzling situation when one thinks about economic security in the region. The dichotomy of prosperity and poverty is a stark reality in South Asia. COVID-19 has been a catastrophe for South Asia largely due to its negative impact on various indicators of economic security in the region. Against this backdrop, some questions are critically important. How does COVID-19 affect economic security in South Asia? What might be the possible policy responses to address the COVID-19 implications on South Asian economic security, both in the short and long terms? This chapter is aimed at investigating these questions with a strong policy focus. It argues that the economic security in South Asia has been affected severely by to the impact of COVID-19.

The chapter is divided into seven sections, including introduction and conclusion. Section 1 introduces the purpose and salient questions of the research while section two theorises economic security to understand the major thrust of impact of COVID-19. The third section dwells on understanding the nature and scope of the economic security of South Asia. The fourth section deals with the relations between COVID-19 and the South Asian economy. The fifth focuses on the implications of COVID-19 for the economic security of South Asia. The sixth section analyses policy responses of South Asia. Finally, the chapter concludes with a futuristic statement.

Theorising Economic Security

Defining economic security is a challenging task as there is a paucity of literature and a contestation about the term 'security'. It is a fact that economic security is linked with a broader understanding of security that captures a central place in international relations scholarship. At its core, security is a relatively simple concept: It refers to safety and survival. Seeking security "involves the pursuit of freedom from threat" (Buzan 1991: 18). Traditionally, it is better understood through questions such as security for whom, security for which values, how much security and from what threats (Baldwin 1997). The question of security for whom indicates a 'referent object'. A referent object may indicate an individual, state, region or international system as actors or climate change, economy or military as issue domains. Security for which values means that actors have values such as physical safety, economic welfare, autonomy, psychological well-being, and so on. How much security implies both absolute and relative conditions. Analysts argue that in a world in which scarce resources must be allocated among competing objectives, none of which is completely attainable, one cannot escape from the question of contentment in attaining security. The final aspect of the question is from what threats does one need to achieve security.

A threat has both subjective and objective dimensions. It can be understood by facts and data such as military strength of adversaries or explicit statements by rival powers. It is also hugely subjective as it involves perception. The so-called 'Soviet threat' or 'communist threat' vs. 'imperialist threat' or 'capitalist threat' during the Cold War era had more subjective elements to understand the magnitude of threat as developed by the two superpowers. However, an assessment of threat is an integral part of understanding security. In this context, threat is always linked with the core values of the referent object. Whatever the sources of threat, it indicates a state of reality in which the core values of actors or issue domains remain safe and preserved (Baldwin 1997). Analysts also indicate that security is a commodity from one perspective; others view it as emancipation (Williams, 2008: 6). Ken Booth (2007:106) has defined security as 'survival plus'. According to Booth, 'The plus here is the choice that comes from (relative) freedom from existential threats'. The relevance of economic security lies with the idea of 'survival plus'.

With this basic understanding of security, it is widely accepted that security has several dimensions or sectors. For instance, Buzan's (1983) *People, States and Fear*, a seminal contribution to the discussion on 'broadening' and 'deepening' security, includes five sectors of security (military, political, economic, societal, and environmental). According to Buzan, economic security is linked with resources, finance, and markets for the purpose of welfare and state power (Williams 2008:4). In another perspective, security has three dimensions—international; economic and human security (Scott et al. 2019: 53). Security is also popularly categorised as traditional security and non-traditional security. Economic security is categorised as non-traditional security.

Scott et al. (2019) argue that economic security is the pursuit of wealth and prosperity. Countries, corporations, and other actors seek wealth and prosperity through profitable economic relations and exchanges; they are ultimately seeking economic security (Scott et al. 2019: 53). Trade competition among countries, cooperation to ensure economic recovery in the wake of the global recession, efforts to deal with debt crises and the ways countries are grappling with the challenges of globalisation signify economic security at the global level (Scott et al. 2019: 53). Gilpin sees economic security from another perspective according to which it is understood as a cause for conflict and war. Gilpin (1981:67) states that 'in a world of scarcity the fundamental issue is the distribution of the available economic surplus', while Stopford and Strange (1991: 204, 209–11) consider the post-cold war era as one characterised by states 'more directly engaged in the competition for shares of the world's wealth'. It is also argued that internal economic dislocation can contribute to conflict for a number of reasons deriving primarily from the pressures that governments find themselves under as a consequence of hard times (Kirshner 2011:278). Economic security is not a new concern for the government, economic instruments being part of the statecraft set for a long time now, a means to influence other states and their policies (Kahler 2004).

Buzan et al. (1998) feel that economic security is located in the intense debates, which regard the relations between the anarchical political structure and the economic structure of the market. Helen E.S. Nesadurai (2005) proposes a comprehensive approach to the concept of economic security to consider socio-economic aspects as well. Another powerful insight about economic security comes from the idea of human security as promoted by the United Nations Development Programme (UNDP) through its famous report titled *The 1994 Human Development Report*. According to the Report,

> The concept of security has for too long been interpreted narrowly: as security of territory from external aggression, or as protection of national interests in foreign policy or as global security from the threat of a nuclear holocaust. It has been related more to nation-states than to people. Forgotten were the legitimate concerns of ordinary people who sought security in their daily lives. For many of them, security symbolised protection from the threat of disease, hunger, unemployment, crime, social conflict, political repression and environmental hazards (UNDP 1994:22).

The UNDP Report (1994) mentions seven specific elements that comprise human security: (1) economic security; (2) food security; (3) health security; (4) environmental security; (5) personal security; (6) community security; and (7) political security. Economic security is the first and foremost pillar of human security that emphasises freedom from poverty. According to the UNDP Report (1994: 25), 'Economic security requires an assured basic income—usually from productive and remunerative work, or in the last resort from some publicly financed safety net. But only about a quarter of the world's people may at present be economically secure in this sense'.

As a synthesis of the scholarly ideas mentioned above, economic security is defined as a situation where the demands of sustainable economic development as means of promoting socio-economic progress at individual and community levels are addressed to ensure peace, freedom and dignity in society. The world as it has evolved since the 1990s demanded a re-definition of what constitutes security. Global developments now suggest the need for another analogous, broadening definition of national security to include resource, environmental and demographic issues (Mathews 2011: 64). Economic security matters because human freedom and dignity matter for every human being. Equally, it should matter for every state in the world. The major thrust of economic security covers several components, which are directly related to alleviate threats to peace, progress, dignity and freedom of human beings. These components include the labour market; employment opportunities; jobs; work; skill development; incomes; distribution and representation.

State of Economic Security in South Asia

South Asia hosts more than a fifth of the world's population and contributes more than 15 per cent of the global economic growth. Since 2014, South Asia has been the fastest-growing sub-region in the world, with its eight economies collectively boosting the average annual growth of 7.0 per cent. This is higher even than East Asia (6.2 per cent), which includes China; Southeast Asia (4.9 per cent); and the Pacific (4.7 per cent) (Song 2011). The IMF (2019) contends that 'South Asia is poised to play a key role in the global economy, building on the steady economic progress and reform process over the last few decades'. It is also argued that 'Despite the recent global economic slowdown, India remains among the fastest-growing large economies, and South Asia's contribution to global growth is set to increase, while those of more mature economies around the world decelerate' (IMF 2019).

Table 2 demonstrates the changes in the economic development of South Asian countries based on the gross domestic product (GDP) at purchasing power parity. All the countries have shown a major rise in their economic progress. Particularly, India and Bangladesh have

Table 1: Basic Indicators of South Asian Countries, 2018

Country	HDI 1990	HDI 2010	HDI 2018	Lifa Expectancy 2018	Mean Years Schooling 2018	$GNI 2018	HDI 2018 Abs Rank	HDI 1990-2018 (%) (Annual Growth)
India	0.431	0.581	0.647	69.4	6.5	6829	8	50.1 (147)
Bangladesh	0.386	0.549	0.614	72.3	6.1	4057	9	59.6 (168)
Pakistan	0.404	0.524	0.56	67.1	5.2	5190	12	38.6 (117)
Nepal	0.380	0.527	0.579	70.5	4.9	2748	11	52.4 (152)
Sri Lanka	0.625	0.75	0.78	76.8	11.1	11,611	2	24.8 (0.08)
Afghanistan	0.298	0.464	0.496	64.5	3.9	1746	13	66.4 (184)

HDI 2010-2018 (%) (Annual Growth)	GNI rank-HDI Rank	Loss in HDI from ineq (%)	National Poverty	Multi-Dim Poverty	Gov. Effectiveness Index 2017	Health Security Index 2019
11.7 (1.36)	−5	26.3	21.9	27.9	0.09	46.5
18.4 (1.41)	6	24.3	24.3	41.7	−0.74	35.0
6.9 (0.83)	−17	31.1	24.3	38.3	−0.58	35.5
9.9 (1.19)	13	25.8	25.2	34.0	−0.38	35.1
4 (0.04)	24	12.1	0.8	0	−0.15	33.9
6.9 (0.83)	1	-	54.5	55.9	−1.33	32.3

Source: Cited in Chhibber (2020).

witnessed a dramatic shift in their economic development. Similarly, Table 2 shows the progress of the region in terms of GDP per capita income.

Table 2: Gross Domestic Product at Purchasing Power Parity (in US$ million)

South Asia	2000	2005	2010	2015	2018
Afghanistan	21,094	26,719	49,145	66,906	76,585
Bangladesh	151,802	214,078	364,054	529,303	704,165
Bhutan	1,615	2,646	4,576	6,514	7,933
India	2,318,667	3,546,543	5,487,141	8,036,327	10,474,334
Maldives	2,179	2,635	4,287	6,162	7,897
Nepal	29,088	38,478	52,569	70,827	86,755
Pakistan	427,259	603,400	715,663	949,730	1,176,498
Sri Lanka	84,781	112,660	168,758	248,090	291,459

Source: Asian Development Bank (2019).

According to the World Economic League Table, Bangladesh has been ranked 41st among the world's largest economies in 2019, which made the country the second-largest economy in South Asia. Among the other South Asian countries, India is ranked 5th, Pakistan 44th, Sri Lanka 66th, Nepal 101st, Afghanistan 115th, the Maldives 156th, and Bhutan 166th (*The Daily Star*, January 8, 2019).

Table 3: Gross Domestic Product per Capita Income (in US$ current)

South Asia	2000	2005	2010	2015	2018
Afghanistan	211	300	657	760	682
Bangladesh	352	416	771	1,224	1,638
Bhutan	738	1,290	2,279	2,721	-
India	475	757	1,435	1,673	2,087
Maldives	2,311	3,436	6,576	9,343	-
Nepal	254	326	620	744	956
Pakistan	565	767	1,006	1,195	1,327
Sri Lanka	863	1,242	2,747	3,845	4,104

Source: Asian Development Bank (2019).

The amazing aspect of economic development in South Asia is observed in the case of sustaining economic growth. Figure 1 shows that during 2000-2018 all the South Asian countries, particularly India, Bangladesh and Nepal, have achieved a major success in GDP growth. Again, Bangladesh and India have registered high growth in the region.

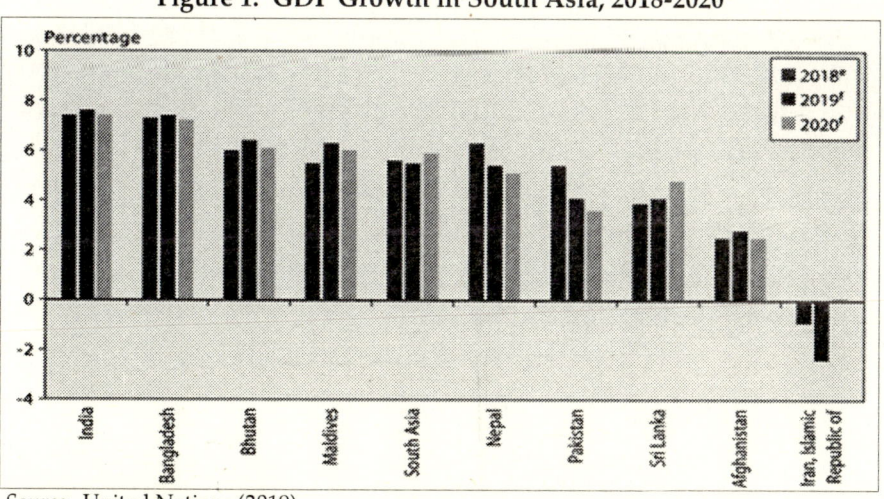

Figure 1: GDP Growth in South Asia, 2018-2020

Source: United Nations (2019).

Based on the macro-level data as mentioned above, the South Asian economic security situation has improved over the last two decades. Particularly, the poverty rate as the major determinant of economic security has witnessed positive changes in the region. As reported by the *Economic Times*, South Asia has made remarkable progress in reducing extreme poverty as compared to the rest of the world. Between 1990 and 2015, the world experienced a 25-percentage point drop in extreme poverty against a 35 percentage-point drop in South Asia (19 September 2018). In fact, the fastest absolute reductions in Multidimensional Poverty Index (MPI) value were in Bangladesh, India, and Cambodia, followed by Ethiopia and Haiti (*The Daily Star*, July 13, 2019).

Threats to Economic Security in South Asia
Despite South Asia performing remarkably well in economic growth and poverty reduction the region remains vulnerable to a number of threats generating economic insecurity for people and communities. These threats or challenges are well addressed in a study titled *South Asia Inequality Report 2019*, conducted by South Asian Alliance for Poverty Eradication (SAAPE). Largely based on the SAAPE report, these are briefly mentioned. First, poverty still remains a number one threat in the whole region. The estimates from the 2018 Global Multidimensional Poverty Index (MPI) released by the United Nations Development Programme (UNDP) and the Oxford Poverty and Human Development Initiative (OPHI) suggest a high incidence of poverty in Nepal (35.3 per cent), Bangladesh (41.1 per cent) and Pakistan (43.9 per cent). Even while India's (27.5 per cent) progress is lauded, it has still a long way to go (SAAPE 2019). South Asia had the second-largest share of the global poor between 1990-2013. It is argued that South Asia's poverty reduction outcomes are negligible compared to East Asia and the Pacific, which were able to lower the share of poor accommodated by 42.9 per cent. Between 2010-2017, the proportion of poor people in South Asia, however, has reduced by 3 per cent while the shares for sub-Saharan Africa and the Arab States have increased by 8 per cent and 2 per cent respectively (Finnigan 2019).

Table 4: Gini Coefficients of South Asian Countries

Country	2009	2010	2011	2012	2013	2014	2015	2016	2017
Afghanistan	-	-	-	27.82	27.82	-	-	31	-
Bangladesh	-	32.1	-	-	-	-	-	32.4	-
Bhutan	-	-	-	38.8	-	-	-	-	37.4
India	-	-	35.1	33.9	33.60	-	35.15	-	-
Maldives	38.4	-	-	-	-	-	-	-	-
Nepal	-	32.8	-	32.82	32.82	32.84	-	-	-
Pakistan	-	29.8	30.9	30.02	30.7	-	33.5	-	-
Sri Lanka	36.4	-	-	39.2	-	-	39.16	39.8	-

Source: UNDP (2009-2017).

Second, inequality continues to characterise economic development in South Asia. The Gini coefficient (Table 4) has increased between 2010 and 2017 in all the eight South Asian countries, which implies that the region as a whole is moving towards greater inequality. As Table 4 shows, the Gini coefficient in Afghanistan has increased from 27.82 in 2012 to 31 in 2016. It has increased from 29.8 in 2010 to 33.5 in 2015 in Pakistan while in Sri Lanka it increased from 36.4 in 2009 to 39.8 in 2016. India has almost the same Gini coefficient between 2011 and 2015. The South Asian population increased by roughly 29 per cent between 2000 and 2017, and the GDP increased by 500 per cent. However, along with this, inequality also increased at a large scale at the same time (SAAPE 2019).

Third, there has been an increasing concentration of wealth in the whole region. No other South Asian country except Bhutan and the Maldives were able to reduce inequality in the years between 1980 to 2015. In India, the top 10 per cent people now hold nearly three-quarters of the total wealth. The top 1 per cent people have been getting richer than the remaining 99 per cent at an unprecedentedly fast pace. In Bangladesh, the income share of the poorest 5 per cent of the population was 0.23 per cent of the overall income, a sharp fall from 2010 when it was 0.78 per cent. In contrast, the share of the income of the richest 5 per cent increased to 27.89 per cent from 24.61 per cent in 2010. In Nepal, the richest 20 per cent of the people have 56.2 per cent of the total wealth while the poorest 20 per cent share only 4.1 per cent of the wealth.

Fourth, landlessness is another chronic feature that poses a constant threat to economic security. Bangladesh has a long history of inequitable access to land; the number of landless households is growing at a fast pace. Thirteen per cent of rural households in Bangladesh own absolutely no type of land, including for housing. In addition, 69.5 per cent rural households lost their land in the past 10 years. In India, as per government estimates, 300 million people are landless in the country. In Pakistan, only 1 per cent of farmland owners (mostly large feudal lords) own 20 per cent of the country's farmland and the top 20 per cent own 69 per cent of the country's farmland.

Fifth, gender inequality remains a significant challenge in South Asia. Women suffer discrimination in the fields of education, health, exposure, employment opportunities and control over resources, and many of them have limited control over their reproductive rights. While, on average globally, women are paid 24 per cent less than men, in South Asia, the gender pay gap is 35 per cent in term of women with children compared to 14 per cent of women without children.

Sixth, South Asia has a growing number of insecure and precarious workers. The high economic growth regime has accelerated informal and unorganised employment, significantly affecting labour market regimes in the region. Uncertain, unstable and insecure employment practices are widely prevalent across the region in addition to rapid informalisation in the formal sector. Out of the total workforce, 90 per cent are in the informal sector in the region. While the number of South Asian billionaires rises at an extremely uncontrollable pace, a vast majority of workers are forced into low-paying jobs with scant or no social protection. Regionally, the rate of informalisation of labour is the highest in India and Nepal (90.7 per cent), with Bangladesh (48.9 per cent), Sri Lanka (60.6 per cent) and Pakistan (77.6 per cent) following.

Seventh, in spite of leaping growth in the number of millionaires and a high GDP, tax collections remain abysmally low in most South Asian countries. In India, the number of people with more than INR 5 million (USD 69,985) income is only 172 thousand, while 12.5 million cars were sold in the years between 2012 and 2017. The number of Indian citizens who flew abroad for either business or tourism, was 20 million in the year 2015. In Pakistan, there was only a minor increase in the tax-to-GDP ratio of 9 per cent (in 2014) to 11.1 per cent in (2018). Bangladesh has one of the lowest tax-to-GDP ratios in the region. In the fiscal year 2016-2017, the tax-to-GDP ratio in Bangladesh was only 9.1 percent, which is far below the developing country average. The South Asian countries are competing with each other to provide the facility of tax exemptions for the rich and the powerful.

Eighth, there is a lack of access to basic services in South Asia in general. The rates of access to infrastructure such as water, sanitation, electricity, telecom and transport in this region are closer to those of Sub-Saharan Africa, the one exception being water. However, there is hardly any city across South Asia that has 24/7 access to water. Despite these problems, the health expenditure in South Asia as a percentage of GDP is terribly low estimated at 3.5 per cent while the global average stands at 10.02 per cent. Over 134 million people still do not have access to improved drinking water in South Asia. Sources of water in South Asia are contaminated, and more than 600 million people in South Asia still practice open defecation (over 60 per cent of the global burden).

Ninth, access to health services in South Asia is very limited. The region faces some of the world's worst socio-economic inequalities, which contribute to one of the worst gaps in access to healthcare facilities. The total government expenditure on healthcare in the region in 2015 was in the range of 0.4-2 per cent of gross domestic product (GDP), which is among the lowest ones globally.

Last, but not least, access to education in the region suffers from resources, misgovernance and rampant privatisation. Only 69 per cent of children have access to early childhood education and only a quarter of young people leave school with the secondary skills they need. In terms of basic literacy rates (for the population of 15 years of age), South Asia lags behind all other regions, except Sub-Saharan Africa, despite the literacy rate rising from 60.84 per cent in 2004 to 71 per cent in 2016.

South Asia falls under one of the regions in the world, which has the lowest public expenditure in education, and that too is diminishing. The lack of public spending on education has adverse impacts on quality education (SAAPE 2019).

As explained above, South Asia has both threats and opportunities in the context of strengthening economic security. Despite facing challenges in poverty reduction, inequality and injustice, South Asia has substantially improved economic conditions over the last two decades. In the wake of the COVID-19 global pandemic, South Asia has emerged as the fastest-growing region in the world. The rise of India and Bangladesh in terms of economic growth drew enormous global attention to the prospects of the whole region as a new centre of prosperity in the world.

COVID-19 and South Asian Economy

The impact of COVID-19 on the South Asian economy is critical to understand how it affects the major indicators of economic security of this region. Although it is a situation in progress, the COVID-19 pandemic is likely to have a damaging economic impact on South Asia, potentially the most serious since the financial crisis two decades ago. A recent World Bank study predicts that South Asia may experience its worst economic performance in 40 years and that half the region could experience a serious recession (Wilson Center 2020). Precisely, in an interconnected and globalised world, the region was thriving on exports of textiles, services and labor to the Middle East and the West. COVID-19 has sparked both a public health emergency and an economic shock in South Asia. South Asia has moved from the fastest-growing region in the world in 2019 to a slow-growth scenario in 2020. Trade, investment and tourism have collapsed. COVID-19 is affecting the global economy, hitting the manufacturing and service sectors alike, with huge impacts on the labour force. The World Bank observes that the current economic conditions in South Asia would be the region's worst performance in the last 40 years, with temporary contractions in all South Asian countries (Figure 2). As played out across the region, the sudden and large-scale loss of low paid work has led to a mass exodus of migrant workers from cities to rural

Figure 2: COVID-19 and GDP Growth Prospects in South Asia

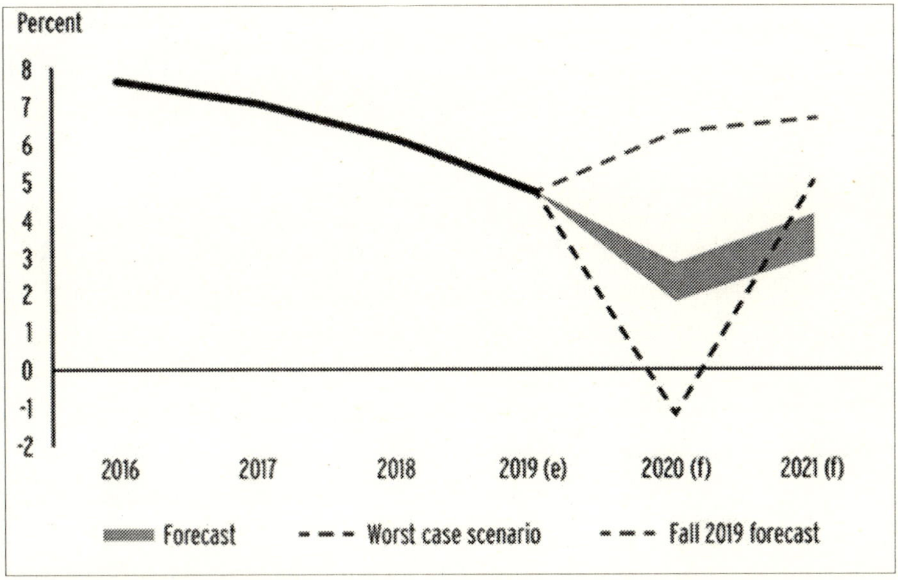

```
Percent
 8
 7
 6
 5
 4
 3
 2
 1
 0
-1
-2
    2016    2017    2018   2019 (e)  2020 (f)  2021 (f)

    ▬▬ Forecast    ▬ ▬ Worst case scenario    ▬ ▬ Fall 2019 forecast
```

Source: Timmer et al. (2020).

areas, spiking the fear that many of them will fall back into poverty (*The Economic Times*, April 12, 2020).

Amitendu Palit at the Institute of South Asian Studies at the National University of Singapore contends that three main factors have created this scenario for South Asia. First, the volume of exports of the South Asian countries will be severely hit as COVID-19 has created a fall in consumption in North America and Europe. It has already affected the economy of Bangladesh and Sri Lanka. Second, job-intensive industries such as tourism, hospitality, civil aviation, retail, construction and housing will be severely affected due to the economic contraction. Third, remittances from the Gulf countries will be affected sharply due to the return of migrant workers (cited in Ovi 2020). Internally, stock markets have tumbled, and business confidence is vanishing. Domestic demand has been reduced dramatically to shutdown and lockdown. Domestic supply chains have been hampered.

The abrupt shutdown of key industries, such as textile production in Bangladesh or the tourism industry in Sri Lanka and the Maldives, will drive up debt and accelerate the threat of recession. The World Bank predicts that 2020 could be the worst business year for South Asia in more than 40 years (Wagner and Scholz 2020). The pandemic is hitting poorer population groups in particular with full force. In India, the unemployment rate had already climbed, by 2019, to its highest level in decades.

In addition, around 90 per cent of all employees in the country work in the in-formal sector. These approximately 450 million people have no social security net whatsoever. After the curfew came into force on March 25, many workers made their way back to their villages. There were also isolated violent clashes with the police. As the states also closed their borders, many migrant workers have been stranded, and their lack of supplies has become a further problem. In general, the region faces major economic stress, collapse of growth, export loss and redirection of global investment. Most significantly, there has been a loss in the gains that South Asia has achieved so far.

Country-wise, while all nations are suffering from the COVID-19 pandemic, some are particularly hard hit. India, as one of the leading global economies in the world, has suffered from both demand and supply shocks. With severe lockdown since the early days of the spread of COVID-19, India became exposed to economic difficulties. One of the major offshoots of lockdown is the migrant crisis, as 80 million internal migrants could not move. It has hampered India's capacity as a food sufficient country due to disruptions at harvest time. India also suffers from disinvestment, loss of revenue, and monetary policy crisis. However, India might attract some investment due to the global mistrust about China.

In Bangladesh, the economic impact has been felt through external and internal shocks. Externally, Bangladesh has already suffered from loss of exports of readymade garment products to Europe and the USA. It is estimated that GDP growth will come down 2-3 per cent, loss of 15 million jobs, deterioration of poverty by an increase to about 40 per cent, loss of revenue and many temporary setbacks in the economy. Hundreds of out-of-work migrant labourers have returned from the Middle East and Europe thus creating a migrant crisis. The Asian Development Bank (ADB) has estimated that Bangladesh will lose about 1.1 per cent of its GDP in the worst-case scenario if the outbreak lasts six months. This means that $3.02 billion from Bangladesh's economy may be lost. Additionally, a global economic downturn may cost Bangladesh 894,930 jobs. Economists estimate that 40 per cent of the total $ 310 billion economy will be exposed to the risks of the pandemic. Bangladesh economy's reliance on remittances, export-oriented readymade garments (RMG) sector, and close trading connections with China make it very vulnerable (Riaz 2020).

For Pakistan, it is a defining moment. Pakistan is facing economic shocks from both demand and supply sides. It also suffers from a loss of export market, job loss, and loss of revenue. Pakistan is particularly vulnerable because of its debt crisis. The country will face more conditionality from the IMF. According to a conservative report, the unemployment rate is projected to surge to 8.1 per cent in the fiscal year 2020-21 (Hasan and Isezaki, 2020). In the case of Afghanistan, the impact is devastating. Food security, loss of domestic revenue (25 per cent down), fiscal crisis, disruption of trade, economic contraction (3-10 per cent for Afghanistan), rising inflation due to high dependence on imported foods (48 per cent for Afghanistan), distributional impacts (high poverty, 55-80 per cent for Afghanistan), disruption of Afghanistan-Pakistan trade, and worsening of poverty in Afghanistan are the key areas of impact.

Thus one can observe that the impact of the COVID-19 pandemic on the South Asian economy is colossal. It has touched upon every aspect of the economy with associated impacts on society, culture, environment, and politics.

Implications for South Asian Economic Security

Having discussed the impact of COVID-19 on South Asian economy, this section directly focuses on the implications for major areas of economic security in the region.

Poverty

The COVID-19 pandemic has a catastrophic impact on vulnerable individuals and households who are already bordering poverty. It may widen inequality gaps and even entrench people in poverty. Daily life has been disrupted, and millions face poverty (Wignaraja et al. 2020). The latest report 'South Asia Economic Focus' anticipates that the COVID-19 pandemic will hit South Asia very hard and the significant gains made in poverty alleviation in the region are likely to be wiped out, the report warned (*The Economic Times*, April 12, 2020). Twenty-three million of the people pushed into poverty are projected to be in Sub-Saharan Africa, and 16 million in South Asia (Mahler et al. 2020).

According to the study of the South Asian Network on Economic Modelling (SANEM), the poverty rate might be back in Bangladesh to a level the country had 15 years ago. Notably, Bangladesh had a poverty rate of 40 per cent in 2005. It is argued that COVID-19 would push Bangladesh's poverty rate to 40.9 per cent, which is exactly the double of the present poverty at 20.5 per cent. In addition to 30.40 million existing poor, and in case of uplifting the poverty line income by 1.25 times, there are another 30.60 million people who are "non-poor" but can be categorised as vulnerable population (cited in *The Business Standard*, May 1, 2020). In the case of India, about 400 million workers in the informal sector would be pushed into deeper poverty due to the impacts of the COVID-19 global pandemic, as claimed by the International Labour Organisation (ILO) (cited in Saini 2020). Shweta Saini (2020) writes in the *Financial Express*,

> ...with the 25% shock to incomes across all fractiles: (i) India's overall poverty rate rises to 46.3%, i.e., more than twice the 2011-12 levels, and higher than even the 1993-94 levels; and (ii) this means that India will have an additional 354 million poor, taking the total count of the country's poor to about 623 million.

Similar trends are expected in other countries of South Asia.

Inequality

Rising inequality poses a substantial hurdle to progress in human development and poverty eradication in South Asia. The COVID-19 pandemic is ruthlessly exposing the gaps between the haves and the have-nots, both within and between countries. South Asia is a region where inequality exists at different levels and sectors. From health to education, from gender to urban-rural level, inequality features prominently, as demonstrated in section three of this chapter. The virus has created a new ground for inequality in the region. Some studies have already pointed out this issue. The primary cause behind this new inequality is the marginalisation of low income and vulnerable people generated through growing staggering joblessness.

According to a World Bank report, low-income people, especially informal workers in the hospitality, retail trade, and transport sectors who have limited or no access to healthcare or social safety nets will be severely affected by the impacts of COVID-19. Inequality in South Asia will increase due to the COVID-19 shock as noted by the report (cited in *The Economic Times*, April 12, 2020). Research on India shows that women are bearing a disproportionate amount of the burden that the imposition of lockdowns and shrinking of economic opportunity has created (Shah 2020). The largest source of inequality in South Asia is access to education, which has been severely disrupted by the pandemic. The existing digital divide in the region has seriously hindered access to education for millions of South Asian students due to the COVID-19 pandemic.

Lives and Livelihoods

The COVID-19 pandemic poses a dilemma for people and nations in South Asia. As seen in other parts of the world, the choice between lives and livelihoods is a stark reality in South Asia where about 1.6 billion work in the informal sectors and more than 80 per cent people live on less than US$ 5.50 a day (Schafer 2018). Although shutdowns and lockdowns have mitigated the spread and saved lives, at the same time, they have also taken away livelihoods. Deepak Nayyer (2020) writes in *The Hindu*,

> In South Asian countries, almost 90% of the workforce is made up of the self-employed, casual labour on daily wages, and informal workers without any social protection. The lockdowns have meant that hundreds of millions of people who have lost their jobs, hence incomes,

have been deprived of their livelihoods, imposing a disproportionate burden on the poor and those who survive just above the poverty line. For them, the trade-off between getting sick and going hungry is no choice. Livelihoods are an imperative for preserving lives.

In the case of Bangladesh, Fahmida Khatun (2020) writes, due to the lockdown in Bangladesh since March 26, 2020, 'informal sector workers—who comprise around 85 per cent of the total workforce—are in dire need of income and food. Preliminary research shows that the daily income of poor people dropped by 76 per cent in the first week of April 2020'. In another development, the Bangladesh readymade garments (RMG) industry received work order cancellations of nearly $3 billion that would affect the livelihoods of around 2 million workers directly engaged with the RMG sector, e.g., backward linkage industries, accessories and packaging factories and transportation sector (Bhuiyan 2020). According to the Bangladesh Sex Workers Network, about 150,000 sex workers in Bangladesh are one of the worst-hit communities following the shutdown (cited in Kepayet 2020). In India, the countrywide lockdown to control the spread of coronavirus has seen 122 million Indians lose their jobs in April alone. According to the Centre for Monitoring the Indian Economy (CMIE), India's unemployment rate is now at a record peak of 27.1 per cent. Asad Umar, the Minister for Planning and Development, Pakistan, notes that around 18 million people might lose their jobs as a result of the lockdown in Pakistan. According to data by the Biruni Institute, six million people have already lost their jobs in Afghanistan due to COVID-19. Notably, 80 per cent people live below the poverty line in the country (cited in Kepayet 2020)

Data from different studies have made it evident that South Asians have been enormously suffering from the loss of livelihoods, which is directly linked with economic security in the region. The governments in South Asia, particularly in Bangladesh, India and Pakistan, have come under sharp criticism for easing lockdowns in some cases and lifting the same in some cases due to the fear of the spread of COVID-19. Simultaneously, the livelihoods of millions of South Asian low wage and informal sector workers are burning issues given the difficult choice of shutdowns and lockdowns. Three issues in this section—poverty, inequality and livelihoods, as analyzed above clearly demonstrate the adverse consequences of the COVID-19 pandemic for the vast majority of the people in South Asia. Besides, a sharp decline in GDP growth, disinvestment, loss of revenue and loss of export markets as direct effects of COVID-19 in South Asia will have a severe impact on the existing socio-economic conditions of people in the region.

Some Positive Trends

While threats to economic security in South Asia are becoming visible in every nation, analysts observe that there is a possibility that South Asia could come through the crisis. One of the strengths of the region is its demography. India, Pakistan and Bangladesh are among the youngest countries in the world, with 5–8 per cent of their populations aged over 60 and 2–3 per cent aged over 70. This compares with Italy's age distribution of about 16 per cent aged over 60, and 10 per cent aged over 70. While there were toilet paper wars that have afflicted Australia's supermarkets, this was not the case for South Asia. There is hardly any report of runs on basic commodities due to COVID-19 (Brewster 2020).

Second, strength of South Asia is social resilience. Though South Asian people have limited resources for social welfare, they have greater social resilience compared to the people in many rich countries. 'People generally rely less on the state and may have more experience in dealing with disasters. Strong social and religious traditions could also provide a valuable reservoir to help resilience' (Brewster 2020).

Third, South Asia, particularly, India and Bangladesh, has experienced relatively high economic growth for several years, that may give an additional advantage to fight against COVID-19.

Fourth, despite endemic food security issues among the poor, exacerbated by recent food price inflation, these countries could be relatively resilient to disruptions in global supply chains. India, Pakistan, and Bangladesh all produce overall food surpluses, helped by high tariff barriers on food imports, which makes them less dependent on global food trade than some other countries. They also have long-established systems for government-supported food distribution to the poor (Brewster 2020).

Fifth, it is also argued that if one looks beyond the present crisis, there lie great opportunities to expand digital technologies for payment systems and distant learning to unlock remote areas in South Asia.

Finally, the strength of the South Asian economy lies in its domestic capacity. It is almost universally recognised that South Asia's economic growth is largely driven by domestic demand and less affected by global economic developments. Domestic demand has increased over the years due to the large development and investment needs. A fast-expanding middle class in the region will also support consumption. The experience of South Asia in facing the 2008-09 global financial crisis bears testimony in this regard.

Policy Responses

Governments in South Asia have responded to this unprecedented crisis by embarking upon a host of new measures. Anticipating potential short and long term economic impacts of COVID-19, governments in India, Pakistan, and Bangladesh have already passed stimulus packages aimed at providing support for the most economically vulnerable in their countries and emergency funding for businesses to weather the current shutdowns. Major thrusts of policy responses in South Asia cover the following:

- Fiscal and monetary stimulus measures—tailored to national circumstances—can mitigate long-term economic damage in South Asia.
- Investing in South Asia's under-developed and over-stretched health systems. As the region lags behind other regions, it must focus on chronic under-spending on public health. For instance, in 2017, South Asia spent only 0.9 per cent of its GDP on public health, which is half the figure for Sub-Saharan Africa (1.9 per cent) and one-fifth of that of East Asia and the Pacific (4.5 per cent) (Wignaraja et al. 2020).

- Livelihood support to vulnerable people, particularly the poorest households, by putting money in their pockets.
- Governments have provided with basic food supplies, either free or at controlled prices, for the poor during lockdowns.
- Incentives for small and medium enterprises (SMEs), garments factories and relevant industries in the form of cash support, reducing tariffs and Customs and taxes.
- Policy support for the recovery of SMEs and creation of jobs.

In Bangladesh, the government has announced a stimulus package for various sectors equivalent to Tk. 964 billion (US$ 11.43 billion), or 3.3 per cent of Bangladesh's GDP. This support is mainly for export-oriented industries, small, medium and large industries, the agriculture sector, pandemic preparations, health workers and social safety net programmes. In India, a large package of stimulus targets almost 800 million people. The Indian government initially made $ 22 billion available to alleviate the economic and humanitarian consequences in the short term, whereas the states initiated their own aid programmes (Wagner 2020). In Pakistan, the government initially provided $ 8 billion to fight the pandemic. As the country currently has double-digit inflation and the IMF did not grant it a rescue package to stabilise the economy until November 2019, Pakistan will have the hardest time obtaining further international aid. The government expects up to 18.5 million people to lose their jobs as a result of the crisis, or more than 30 per cent of the work-force. Another measure has been to expand social programmes such as the Benazir Income Support Programme (Wagner 2020).

As far as post COVID-19 policies are concerned, the Government of India has initiated several measures: (a) Self-reliance in the Indian economy as the key forte; (b) new modes of industries to develop the Indian economy from a new angle; (c) emphasis on the development of manufacturing sectors; (d) innovations of new updated technology along with skilled manpower; (e) pivotal roles of private sector banks; (f) cash transfer to the innumerable migrant labourers as well as for the poor and downtrodden; and (g) emphasis upon the development of cottage and small scale industries along with agro-based industries (Das 2020). Similarly, in the case of Bangladesh, policy measures include: (i) speedy completion of Metro Railway projects with the cooperation of China and Japan; (ii) maintaining friendship with India as a key factor to deal with post-COVID economic challenges; (iii) stepping up the development of garment industries; and (iv) aggressive cash transfer should be done by the government of Bangladesh like India for the betterment of migrant labourers as well as for the betterment of the poor and downtrodden (Das 2020).

Considering the unique nature of South Asian economic security, the governments will make efforts for debt cancellation, which will strengthen their public health system, for example, staffing, medical equipment, medicine stock, infrastructure, research, production of medicines, etc. South Asia, in general, and India in particular, is also eyeing a redirection of investment from China in the post-COVID-19 era.

Conclusion

This chapter has argued that the COVID-19 global pandemic has exacerbated the existing threats to economic security in South Asia. Shocks from both supply and demand sides have significantly threatened people's lives and the region's economic outlook. Besides, it has created an unprecedented and new ground for exploiting the poor and the most vulnerable sections of society in South Asia. It further argues that due to the unique nature of the South Asian economy, which is widely marked by informalisation and local resources, people are facing more challenges in coping with the COVID-19 crisis. A critical issue is that although South Asian countries have substantially liberalised their economies that have increased their dependence on growth and corporate expansion, the immediate policy responses of the governments during the COVID-19 crisis should prioritise people over economic recovery. Large fiscal measures, monetary policy, development priorities and economic recovery strategies should be focused on the long term goal of bringing back high GDP growth in the region as already forecast by the World Bank.

However, without due attention to the sources of economic insecurity in South Asia, no sustainable progress will be achieved. In this context, a host of issues need urgent consideration to both policy and academic community. First, the local disruptions of economic and financial systems, the plausibility of overall economic and the financial crisis must be tackled. Second, standards of living as indicators of economic security—overlaps with human security—should be highlighted in policymaking. Third, corruption, irregularities and other illicit economic activities in the region must be considered security threats. Fourth, poverty, inequality and distributive injustice stemming from a singular focus on economic growth should be addressed during and after the COVID-19 crisis. The demographic patterns in South Asia should be a major determinant of policy choice in the economic development agenda. Fifth, environmental consequences are vital to understand the quality of life in the region marked by an acute level of air pollution, climate change and other sources of environmental degradation. Sixth, integration with the global economy through investment, trade, aid, technology and knowledge should be refocused in such as a way that addresses the threats to economic security in the region. Finally, South Asian people and governments must take the leverage within the region and beyond for its great advantages of having a youthful population, a growing middle-class and a strategic geographical location

REFERENCES

Asian Development Bank (2019). *Key Indicators for Asia and the Pacific.* Manila: ADB.

Aneez, S. & Saif, S. K. (2020, April 29). 'Should I buy a mask or food?': South Asia's poor face stark choice. *The Japan Times.* Retrieved from https://www.japantimes.co.jp/news/2020/04/29/asia-pacific/social-issues-asia-pacific/mask-or-food-south-asia-poor/#.XvLImBJS_IV

Baldwin, D.A. (1997). The concept of security. *Review of International Studies,* 23(1), 5-26.

Bhuiyan, M. S. A. (2020, April 15). COVID-19 and its impact on Bangladesh economy. *The Business Standard.* Retrieved from https://tbsnews.net/thoughts/COVID-19-and-its-impact-bangladesh-economy-69541

Booth, K. (2007). *Theory of world security.* New York: Cambridge University Press.

Brewster, D. (2020, April 10). Why South Asia may come out of COVID-19 crisis better than many expect. *The Interpreter.* Retrieved from https://www.lowyinstitute.org/the-interpreter/why-south-asia-may-come-out-COVID-19-crisis-better-many-expect

Buzan, B. (1983). *People, states and fear: National security problem in International Relations*, Sussex: Wheatsheaf Books Ltd.

Buzan, B. (1987). *An introduction to Strategic Studies: Military technology and International Relations* (London: Macmillan).

Buzan, B. (1991). *People, states and fear: An agenda for International Security Studies in the post-Cold War era* (London: Harvester Wheatsheaf, 2nd edn).

Buzan, B. (1997). Rethinking security after the end of the Cold War. *Cooperation and Conflict.* 32(1), 5-28.

Buzan, B., Ole Wæver, O. & Jaap de Wilde, J. d. (1998). *Security: A new framework for analysis.* Boulder, CO: Lynne Rienner.

Chhibber, A. (2020, April 4). A new "Asian drama": Will COVID-19 destroy the progress against poverty eradication and human development in South and East Asia?. Atlantic Council. Retrieved from https://www.atlanticcouncil.org/blogs/new-atlanticist/a-new-asian-drama-will-COVID-19-destroy-the-progress-against-poverty-eradication-and-human-development-in-south-and-east-asia/

Das, S. (2020, May 18). The economic impact of COVID-19 on South Asia. *The Daily Asian Age.* Retrieved from https://dailyasianage.com/news/229765/the-economic-impact-of-COVID-19—on-south-asia

Finnigan, C. (2019, April 9). Poverty in South Asia; The long view. LSE Blogs. Retrieved from https://blogs.lse.ac.uk/southasia/2019/04/09/poverty-in-south-asia-the-long-view/

Gilpin, R. (1981) *War and Change in World Politics.* Cambridge: Cambridge University Press.

Hasan, M. & Isezaki, K. (2020, April 30). *Challenges for South Asia in, and after, pandemic: The primacy of politics in the region will require radical reform to cope with the post-COVID-19 world. Asia Times.* Retrieved from https://asiatimes.com/2020/04/challenges-for-south-asia-in-and-after-pandemic/

IMF (2019, November 4). Building on South Asia's economic success. Retrieved from https://www.imf.org/en/News/Articles/2019/11/01/NA110219-building-on-south-asias-economic-success

Kahler, M. (2004). Economic security in an era of globalization: definition and provision, *The Pacific Review,* 17(4), 485-502, DOI: 10.1080/0951274042000326032

Kepayet, M. (2020, May 20). Job loss, hunger stalk South Asia in COVID-19 times. *South Asia Monitor.* Retrieved from https://southasiamonitor.org/spotlight/job-loss-hunger-stalk-south-asia-COVID-19-times

Khatun, F. (2020, May 7). COVID-19 batters Bangladesh's already struggling economy. *East Asia Forum.* Retrieved from https://www.eastasiaforum.org/2020/05/07/COVID-19-batters-bangladeshs-already-struggling-economy/

Kirshner, J. (2011). Economics and security. In C. W. Hughes and L.Y. Meng (eds.), *Security studies: A reader* (pp. 278-292). Abingdon, Oxon and New York: Routledge.

Mahler, D.G., Lakner, C., Aguilar, R.A.C. & Wu, H. (2020, April 20). The impact of COVID-19 (Coronavirus) on global poverty: Why Sub-Saharan Africa might be the region hardest hit. World Bank Blogs. Retrieved from https://blogs.worldbank.org/opendata/impact-COVID-19-coronavirus-global-poverty-why-sub-saharan-africa-might-be-region-hardest

Mathews, J. T. (2011). Redefining security (2). In C. W. Hughes and L.Y. Meng (eds.),

Security studies: A reader (pp.64-70). Abingdon, Oxon and New York: Routledge.

Nayyer, D. (2020, April 24). The COVID-19 paradox in South Asia. *The Hindu*. Retrieved from https://www.thehindu.com/opinion/lead/the-COVID-19-paradox-in-south-asia/article31417806.ece

Nesadurai, H.E.S. (2005). Conceptualising economic security in an era of globalisation: What does the East Asian experience reveal?. CSGR Working Paper No. 157/05, Centre for the Study of Globalisation and Regionalisation (CSGR), University of Warwick, Coventry. Retrieved from http://www2.warwick.ac.uk/fac/soc/csgr/research/workingpapers/2005/wp15705.pdf

Ovi, I. H. (2020, May 16). Economists: Labour market, poverty major challenges in post-Coronavirus era. *Dhaka Tribune*. Retrieved from https://www.dhakatribune.com/business/economy/2020/05/16/economists-labour-market-poverty-major-challenges-in-post-coronavirus-era

Raihan, S. (2020, April 9). Case for a united South Asian response to COVID-19. *The Daily Star*. Retrieved from https://www.thedailystar.net/opinion/news/case-united-south-asian-response-COVID-19-1891000

Riaz, A. (2020, March 31). Bangladesh. South Asia's economic outlook in the era of COVID-19. Atlantic Council Blogs. Retrieved from https://www.atlanticcouncil.org/blogs/new-atlanticist/south-asias-economic-outlook-in-the-era-of-COVID-19/

Saini, S. (2020, April 30). COVID-19 may double poverty in India. *The Financial Express*, India. Retrieved from https://www.financialexpress.com/opinion/COVID-19-may-double-poverty-in-india/1943736/

Scott, J.M., Ralph G. Carter, R.G. & Drury, A.C. (2019). *IR: national, international economic and human security in a changing world*. London: Sage/CQ Press.

Schafer, H. (2018, October 17). Finishing job of ending poverty in South Asia. The World Bank Blogs. Retrieved from https://blogs.worldbank.org/endpovertyinsouthasia/finishing-job-ending-poverty-south-asia

Shah, K. (2020, May 17). How COVID-19 is amplifying gender inequality in India. *The Indian Express*. Retrieved from https://indianexpress.com/article/opinion/coronavirus-gender-inequality-india-6414659/

Song, L. L. (2019, August 4). How South Asia can continue as world's fastest growing subregion. *Modern Diplomacy*. Retrieved from https://moderndiplomacy.eu/2019/08/04/how-south-asia-can-continue-as-worlds-fastest-growing-subregion/

South Asia Alliance for Poverty Eradication (SAAPE) (2019). *Growing Inequality in South Asia: South Asian Inequality Report 2019*, Kathmandu: SAAPE.

Stopford, F. &, Strange, S. (1991). *Rival States Rival Firms: Competition for World Market Shares*. Cambridge: Cambridge University Press.

Timmer, H., Mercer-Blackman, V. & Beyer, R.C.M. (2020, April 16). The economic impact of COVID-19 on South Asia: 3 Visuals. World Bank Blogs. Retrieved from https://blogs.worldbank.org/endpovertyinsouthasia/economic-impact-COVID-19-south-asia-3-visuals

The Business Standard (2020, May 1). COVID-19 impacts may double poverty in Bangladesh, says think tank. Retrieved from https://tbsnews.net/economy/COVID-19-impacts-may-double-poverty-bangladesh-says-think-tank-76027

The Daily Star (2019, January 8). Bangladesh 2nd largest economy in South Asia.

Retrieved from https://www.thedailystar.net/bangladesh/bangladesh-ranked-41st-largest-economy-in-2019-all-over-the-world-study-1684078

The Economic Times (2018, September 19). Pace of extreme poverty reduction in S Asia faster than rest of the world: World Bank. Retrieved from https://economictimes.indiatimes.com/news/international/business/pace-of-extreme-poverty-reduction-in-s-asia-faster-than-rest-of-the-world-world-bank/articleshow/65875618.cms?utm_source=contentofinterest&utm_medium=text&utm_campaign=cppst

The Economic Times (2020, April 12). COVID-19 to hit South Asia very hard, likely to wipe out gains made in poverty alleviation: World Bank. Retrieved from https://economictimes.indiatimes.com/news/economy/finance/COVID-19-to-hit-south-asia-very-hard-likely-to-wipe-out-gains-made-in-poverty-alleviationworld-bank/articleshow/75104473.cms?utm_source=contentofinterest&utm_medium=text&utm_campaign=cppst

UNDP (1994). *Human development report 1994*. New York: Oxford University Press.

UNDP (2009-2017). *Human development report 2009-2017*. New York: Oxford University Press.

United Nations (2019). *World Economic Situation and Prospects 2019*. New York: United Nations.

Wagner, C. & Tobias Scholz, T. (2020, April). South Asia in the Corona Crisis: Economic and political consequences. SWP Comment 2020/C 19, 4 Pages. Retrieved from https://www.swp-berlin.org/10.18449/2020C19/

Wignaraja, G., Raihan, S., Sharma, P., Ahmed, V. & De, P. (2020, April 26). Five Proposals to Tackle COVID-19 in South Asia. *The Prospector*. Retrieved from https://lki.lk/blog/five-proposals-to-tackle-COVID-19-in-south-asia/

Williams, P.D. (2008). Security Studies: An introduction. In P.D. Williams (ed.), *Security Studies: An Introduction* (pp. 1-12), New York: Routledge.

Wilson Center (2020, May 14). Webcast: Economic Implications of COVID-19 for South Asia. Retrieved from https://www.wilsoncenter.org/event/webcast-economic-implications-COVID-19-south-asia

5

Environmental Security in South Asia

ABSTRACT

What are the implications of COVID-19 for environmental security in South Asia about air pollution, and climate change? What would be the policy imperatives? This chapter investigates these questions. Though the COVID-19 global pandemic created some negative consequences for humans, it has been a blessing for the environment. Due to lockdown measures and business closures, there is a significant reduction in carbon emissions, both regionally and globally. Air pollution has been reduced significantly in South Asia. This chapter argues that the COVID-19 global pandemic is a wake-up call to save the global environment from imminent destruction. It becomes of paramount interest to ensure clear air and address global climate change for the sustainable environmental security of the people in South Asia and beyond. It is also critically important to nurture cognitive awareness derived from the COVID-19 global pandemic for a sustainable planet. Thus, this chapter suggests taking a lesson from COVID-19 and maintaining a healthy balance between corporate profits and the environment for the enhancement of environmental security.

Keywords: *COVID-19, Environmental Security, Air Pollution, Climate Change, Carbon Emission, South Asia.*

Introduction

The twenty-first century is called the age of Anthropocene, a new geological epoch. The popular discourse is that human actions, the capitalist economic system, the capitalist way of living, economic accelerations, over-extraction of resources, waste dumping are contributing to changing the earth system (Hamilton et al. 2015). It is called a new epoch where unprecedented levels of global warming and climate change, ocean acidification, biodiversity loss have become a common phenomenon. Ecological unsustainability defines this new epoch of Anthropocene. It is argued that the first stage of Anthropocene started between 1750 and 1800 when humans began to use energy, fossil fuels. The second stage of Anthropocene began in 1950 with the rapid economic accelerations, with the increased level use of carbon emissions, depletion of ozone. It is manifest that certain actors, i.e., the corporate world, have concentrated on profit maximising activities throughout centuries at the expense of the global environment. In fact, in the pursuit of economic growth, the developed countries through industrial revolutions have made the world inhabitable through polluting the global environment. Thus, it was essential to rethink the sustainability of the planet. In fact, the COVID-19 global pandemic has brought a blessing for the global environment by reducing the carbon emissions, improving air quality.

Return of clear skies along with a decline in global carbon emissions has been the concrete, visible positive outcomes of the COVID-19 global pandemic. In fact, lockdown measures to contain the novel coronavirus have curtailed human activities both in the ocean and land and have resulted in such a positive outcome. This outcome has not been observed for many decades. After the Second World War, there was no instance of global carbon emission decline in such a level/rate. Air traffic, traffic on the surface/roads have also been reduced significantly in the lockdown days. Thus carbon dioxide, carbon oxides, nitrogen oxides, sulphur oxide emissions have been reduced, which has had a positive impact on the overall environment. Air quality has been improved globally, including in South Asia. The COVID-19 global pandemic has brought an opportunity to rethink about maintaining a balance between human need, greed, and the global environment.

It is also noticed that marine life is in the process of recovery as there are reduced pressures on stocks due to the COVID-19 global pandemic. It is seen that dolphins are dancing in the sea off Mumbai, Cox's Bazar and other beaches in South Asia (*Times of India*, March 24, 2020; Lipu 2020). Thus, it is argued that 'Coronavirus lockdowns globally have given parts of the natural world a rare opportunity to experience life' (*BBC News*, April 29, 2020). Bhutto Khan, a regular surfer on the Cox's Bazar sea beach, points out that 'Suddenly, the dolphins have come very close to the beach. We did not see this in the past' (quoted in Lipu 2020). Kabir Ahmed, an oyster seller for 25 years in Cox's Bazar sea beach, notes that 'I saw sea oysters, snails, red crabs, and sea creepers some 15-20 years ago. I thought they had become extinct. But I am very happy to see them again' (quoted in Lipu 2020). A considerable number of nomadic crabs are returned in Kuakata sea beach, Bangladesh, which had disappeared due to indiscriminate human activities (Hossain 2020). One can argue that if human activities in the ocean could be controlled, marine bio-diversity could be rejuvenated. Additionally, the closures of restaurants and hotels and the difficulties in maintaining social distancing among crews at sea have halted marine fishing as the two World Wars did. Duarte contends that 'Studies after the first and second world wars showed a spectacular recovery. We are hoping that this unintended closed season between February and June or July will accelerate the recovery of fish stocks and allow us to reach conservation objectives faster' (cited in *The Japan Times*, April 18, 2020). Thus, one can argue that the COVID-19 global pandemic has substantial implications for the overall environment in South Asia. Among the different environmental dimensions, this chapter focuses on air pollution and climate change with case studies to understand the implications of COVID-19 for South Asian environmental security.

This chapter is divided into six sections, including the introduction and conclusion. The background and research questions of the chapter are discussed in the introduction section. The second section explains the environmental challenges in South Asia, while the third section examines COVID-19 impacts on air pollution and climate change in South Asia. The fourth section focuses on COVID-19 implications on South Asian environmental security, while the fifth section deals with policy imperatives. The final section concludes.

Conceptualising Environmental Security

For long, security has been seen through the lenses of the state, i.e., national security. Here, the referent object of security has been identified as states, which are concerned about ensuring territorial integration by military means. This is also known as traditional security. However, due to the end of the Cold War, and the changing nature of security threats, the concept of security has been problematised, broadened, and deepened. Thus, there were scholarly attempts to redefine security, including environmental components (Buzan 1983; Mathews 1989; Booth 1991; Homer-Dixon 1991). It is argued that the concept of environmental security 'has been developed as an alternative to the traditional concept of security. The discussion on the concept of environmental security has concentrated on the unit of analysis: it has been suggested that an environmental component be included in the concept of national security, global security or societal security' (Tennberg 1995:239).

Thomas Homer-Dixon (1991, 1994) is one of the most prominent scholars in the field of environmental security. Homer-Dixon prefers the term 'environmental scarcity' instead of 'environmental security'. Environmental resource scarcity has been identified as a source of conflicts. Homer-Dixon (1991) contends that simple scarcity conflicts can be explained by general structural theories that posit that external constraints can encourage or even compel actors to engage in conflict. Domestic structural theories view that organised groups within a society can spark conflicts through articulating, channelling, and coordinating discontents. According to Homer-Dixon (1991), simple scarcity conflicts arise over three types of resources, i.e., river water, fish, and agriculturally productive land. These resources are essential for human survival and thus spark conflicts. These resources can also be physically seized or controlled. Thus, it can also create inter-group and inter-state simple-scarcity conflicts or resource wars (Homer-Dixon 1994:6).

In fact, defining the concept of environmental security is seen as a 'risky business' (Tennberg 1995) and contested with various meanings. It is seen as an 'elusive' concept (Ney 1999). It has been defined both from national and human security perspectives. The proponents of national security are mainly concerned with the question of how national security can be threatened by environmental changes while human security proponents mainly deal with the question of how human security can be threatened by environmental changes. From the perspective of national security, Braden R. Allenby (2000:5) defines environmental security as 'the intersection of environmental and national security considerations at a national policy level'.

'Environmental security' within the domain of human security has been popularised by the publication of a UNDP 1994 report. In the domain of environmental security, the UNDP report identifies the issue of water scarcity, land shortage, air pollution, and natural disasters as environmental threats faced by both developing and developed states. From a human security perspective, Barnett et al. (2010:18) define environmental security as: 'When people do not have enough options to avoid or to adapt to environmental change such that their needs, rights, and values are likely to be undermined, then they can be said to be environmentally insecure'. Additionally, from a human security perspective, environmental security can be defined as safety from 'Threats to a productive, healthy life due to environmental factors such as natural disasters, poor resource management, and climate change' (Saferworld 2008:13).

For Peter Hough (2019:1) 'From either a human or national security perspective environmental security emerged as a concept from the 1990s intended to signify a heightened significance for issues of environmental change beyond that already apparent in the politicisation of nature inherent in the rise of political ecology'. However, this chapter uses environmental security from the perspective of human security, focusing broadly on human well-being.

Key Environmental Challenges in South Asia

South Asia is often cited as the most vulnerable region in the context of global warming and climate change. Natural disasters are frequent in the region. Though most of the South Asian countries contribute less to global warming and climate change, they are most vulnerable to its impacts. Among environmental challenges, climate change, air pollution, water pollution, soil degradation, marine plastic pollution, deforestation is notable. Some of the key environmental challenges are discussed here.

Air Pollution

Air pollution is a mixture of solid particles and gases in the air. Some air pollutants are poisonous, and inhaling it can cause different diseases. The World Health Organisation (WHO) notes that 'Ambient (outdoor air pollution) is a major cause of death and disease globally. The health effects range from increased hospital admissions and emergency room visits to increased risk of premature death' (WHO, n.d.). Thus, improved air quality becomes essential for health benefits (Tian et al. 2020). According to a 2019 report by Swiss air quality technology company IQAir, India, Bangladesh, and Pakistan are among the most polluted in the world (cited in *Himal South Asian*, April 22, 2020). Dhaka is the second most polluted capital city after Delhi. Notably, 22 out of the top 30 polluted cities are located in India (Molla, 2019). According to the WHO, 10 out of the 11 most polluted cities are in India (Chandrasekaran 2019). Kabul is one of the most polluted cities in the world (*Al Jazeera*, January 16, 2019). In this chapter, we focus on the air pollution challenge in South Asia by looking at its impacts on economic growth and diseases.

There is a strong linkage between economic growth and air pollution and vice versa. On one hand, the neo-liberal economic model based on the 'profits over people' principle leads to increasing use of fossil fuels resulting in air pollution at a severe level. Thus, increasing air pollution has contributed to health risks to urban citizens, mainly. On the other hand, air pollution has severe economic implications, which ultimately affect the overall human security of the people in South Asia. For instance, if a large (productive) section of people become affected by an infectious disease like novel coronavirus, it can create a disastrous situation for the productivity of South Asian nations. Also, air pollution hampers the achieving of the full potential of the people in the region, which becomes an impediment for the overall socio-economic development of South Asian nations. One also needs to note that the people affected by different air pollution-related diseases need to spend large amounts of money for medical treatment. Thus, poor people in the region are severely affected. Additionally, it is claimed that due to air pollution, India loses US$ 150 billion annually, while Bangladesh loses US$ 14 billion (Farrow et al. 2020). The economic loss from air pollution for other South Asian countries is also high (Table 1).

Table 1: Impact Attributed to Fossil Fuel-related Air Pollution in South Asia (Estimated total cost in million USD)

Country	Low	Central	High
Afghanistan	170	270	380
Bangladesh	9,100	14,000	18,000
Bhutan	31	54	79
India	100,000	150,000	190,000
Maldives	17	26	38
Nepal	580	940	1400
Pakistan	3,800	6,100	9,200
Sri Lanka	460	760	1100

Source: Farrow et al. 2020: 29-35.

One cannot deny that for South Asian countries, where human development indicators are not satisfactory, this massive amount of money could be invested in the social development sector. According to UNECE (n.d.), air pollution 'takes its toll of the economy in several ways: It costs human lives, it reduces people's ability to work, it affects vital products like food, it reduces the ability of ecosystems to perform functions societies need, and it costs money in remediation or restoration'. One can also argue that if air pollution is not controlled, even other administrative functions will collapse (during the winter season, especially) in cities like Delhi or Dhaka in the coming decades. For instance, in April 2015, *The Indian Express* reported that doctors are suggesting to patients with serious respiratory ailments to leave Delhi (Chatterjee, April 2, 2015). If the working force has to leave the capital, it will bring disastrous consequences for the economic activities of South Asian countries. Additionally, diseases from air pollution can turn a vibrant city like Dhaka or Delhi into a ghost city. In this link, one can mention the coronavirus impact on European or North American cities.

It is a well-known fact that air pollution causes various diseases. In this regard, Dr. Mrinal Sircar, director and head, Department of Pulmonology & Critical Care, Fortis Hospital, Noida, said that air pollution increases the risk of lung cancer, respiratory and heart diseases, asthma problems (*The Indian Express*, June 5, 2019). Breathing in polluted air decreases the lung functions which can also cause chronic obstructive pulmonary disease (COPD) according to a study of Anna Hansell, a professor at the University of Leicester, UK (*The Indian Express*, July 10, 2019). COPD is a long-term process and is the third leading cause of death worldwide, which might increase in the next ten years, according to the Global Burden Project (*The Indian Express*, July 10, 2019). Hansell contends that 'Worryingly, we found that air pollution had much larger effects on people from lower-income households' (cited in *The Indian Express*, July 10, 2019). Additionally, one can ask how many poor people in the region would be able to buy air purifiers. The day is not so far when pure air will be sold in the market like bottled mineral water. It is also assumed that the price will certainly be very costly for the poor. Thus, the poor section in society becomes the most vulnerable to air pollution.

One also needs to look at the impact of air pollution on children. Children are the future of South Asia. Though everyone is affected by air pollution, children from 0 to 10 years are most vulnerable (Chandrasekaran 2019). The UN health body claims that 93 per cent of children (under the age of 15) breathe dangerously polluted air every day (*Dhaka Tribune*, April 3, 2019). Additionally, researchers from the University of Cincinnati and Cincinnati Children's Hospital Medical Centre in the USA find that traffic air pollution increases the risk of childhood mental disorders, i.e., anxiety and depression (*The Indian Express*, May 23, 2019). This applies in the case of South Asian countries. According to UNICEF, 'South Asia has the largest proportion of babies under the age of one living in the worst-affected areas, with 12.2 million babies residing where outdoor air pollution exceeds six times international limits set by the World Health Organisation (WHO)' (UN Sustainable Development Goals Blog, December 6, 2017).

Climate Change

While the whole world is concerned about the number of infected, deaths, impacts, and vaccines of COVID-19, the fact that super cyclone Amphan (May 2020) destroyed tens of thousands of houses, roads, culverts, damaged crops, and caused about 100 deaths in Bangladesh and India underscores the vulnerability of South Asia to climate change as well as the urgency to resolve climate disasters. In fact, one needs to acknowledge that climate change is the greatest environmental challenge South Asia is facing today. Though the contribution of the South Asian countries to global warming and climate change is very negligible, they are the most vulnerable countries to climate change. For instance, Bangladesh is identified on the 'frontline of climate emergency' (Marsh 2020). The location of the South Asian countries makes them the most disaster-prone countries in the world. Thus, natural disasters like cyclones, tropical storms, floods are a common phenomenon in South Asia due to the location and impacts of climate change. It is noted that 'In the past decade alone, nearly 700 million people—half of the region's population—were affected by one or more climate-related disasters' (Fallesen et al. 2019). It is estimated that the damage caused by disasters between 2000 and 2017 was worth US$ 149.27 billion. Notably, between 1990 and 2008, natural disasters caused 230,000 deaths in South Asia (Ahmed and Suphachalasai 2014).

It is expected that 800 million people in the region will be severely affected by the impact of climate change, which will burden the South Asian economy (Fallesen et al. 2019). By 2030, according to the World Bank, 62 million people in South Asia will be pushed below the poverty line by the impacts of climate change (cited in Fallesen et al. 2019). Without substantial global action, global temperature may rise by 4.6°C, which will affect the South Asian economy badly. The economy of Bangladesh, Bhutan, India, the Maldives, Nepal, and Sri Lanka could shrink by up to

1.8 per cent every year by 2050 and 8.8 per cent by 2100, on an average (Ahmed and Suphachalasai 2014).

Filippo Grandi, the United Nations High Commissioner for Refugees, contends that the world needs to prepare for millions of climate refugees (*Al Jazeera*, January 21, 2020). Nidhi Adlakha (2020) writes that 'climate crisis is creating more refugees than war'. South Asia might experience millions of climate refugees shortly. In this regard, Atiq Rahman, Executive Director, Bangladesh Centre for Advanced Studies, notes that by 2070-90, half of the coastal districts of Bangladesh will disappear due to the impact of climate change (*The Daily Star*, April 24, 2018). Sheikh Hasina, the Prime Minister of Bangladesh, pointed out in Parliament that around 40 million people from 19 coastal districts might be displaced due to the impact of climate change (*The Daily Star*, January 15, 2020). There are huge negative consequences, including loss of lives, livelihood, and infrastructure due to natural disasters.

One also needs to think about the impact of climate change on the rising sea level in South Asia, especially in low-lying Bangladesh. According to the Climate Smart Agriculture Investment Plan (CSAIP) Bangladesh, 'With two-thirds of the country at an elevation of less than 5 metres, Bangladesh is highly exposed to rising sea-levels, particularly the southern region. Rising sea levels and salinisation are already being felt across coastal areas' (*The Daily Star*, December 12, 2019). Mahfuz Ahmed, principal climate change specialist with ADB's South Asia Department, notes that loss of snow cover in the Himalayas and sea-level rise threatens the livelihoods of more than 200 million people in Bangladesh, Bhutan, the Maldives, Nepal, and Sri Lanka (ADB 2013). Therefore, the impact of climate change in South Asia is severe from multiple dimensions, which affect environmental security for the South Asian people. This merits serious attention, both from policy and academic inquiry.

Marine Plastic Pollution

Marine plastic pollution is another severe environmental challenge for South Asia yet understudied. In fact, the title of Pennington's article, i.e.,

'Every minute, one garbage truck of plastic is dumped into our oceans. This has to stop' underscores the severity of plastic pollution in the oceans as well as a call for ending this (Pennington, 2016). According to a study by Jenna Jambeck and her colleagues of the University of Georgia, every year, 8 million metric tons of plastic that are produced by 192 coastline states enter the oceans (Schupska, 2015). One can imagine how much plastics has been dumped into the oceans over the years, over the decades. Marine plastic pollution was first reported in scientific literature in the early 1970s (Schupska 2015) though it has been happening for centuries. In fact, if such dumping continues, it is argued that there will be more plastic than fish in the oceans by 2050 (Pennington, 2016). UN oceans chief Lisa Svensson defines the plastic pollution in oceans as a 'planetary crisis' (Harrabin, 2017). This marine plastic pollution has been a grave concern for marine life over the decades. In the case of the Bay of Bengal, Bangladesh alone contributes to about 2 lakh tons of plastics every year (Islam 2019). In a survey, 2,619 pieces of plastics are found in a 5.5 km sea beach in Bangladesh (Amin 2018). Among the top 15 countries that produced the most plastic waste in 2010, Sri Lanka was ranked 5th, Bangladesh 10th, India 12th, and Pakistan was ranked 15th position (Harrabin 2017). Against this backdrop, this chapter argues that marine plastic pollution needs to be controlled to ensure a sustainable ocean for our common future. The ten rivers that contribute to 90 per cent of ocean plastic pollution, two (i.e., Ganga and Indus) are shared by the South Asian states (*Sky News*, December 12, 2017). There are a number of negative consequences of marine plastic pollution for marine life and marine biodiversity. Mehedi Al Amin writes that 'Plastic lasts up to 1,000 years, and accounts for nearly 90 per cent of the debris in the oceans around the world. Plastic also kills up to one million sea birds and 100,000 sea mammals and countless fish every year' (Amin, 2018). It becomes pertinent to mention that in June 2018, a whale died off Thailand; it had 80 plastic bags in its stomach (*BBC*, 2018). In March 2019, another dead whale was found in the Philippines with 88 pounds of plastic trash in its stomach (Victor, 2019). Thus, one can understand the severity of marine plastic pollution, which works as one of the key environmental challenges for South Asia.

Soil Degradation

Esther Ngumbi (2020) writes in Project Syndicate that 'Soils are strategic assets that underpin agriculture, farm productivity, and national economies, yet they are suffering widespread damage, erosion, drying, and degradation. It is high time we reversed this trend'. Soil degradation is another critical environmental challenge for South Asia. Soil is one of the most important natural resources that constitute the very basis of human life. Soil degradation, including soil erosion, has been a common phenomenon in South Asian countries. Myers (1989:23) writes that 'The effects of soil erosion on agricultural productivity are a legitimate cause for international concern, whether the erosion occurs in India or in Indiana'. It is noted that 42 per cent of South Asia's land is affected by various forms of degradation (Singh and Singh 2011). Abul Kalam Azad (2011), director of SAARC Agriculture Centre, notes that water erosion affects about eighty-three million hectares of land in South Asia. Wind erosion affects 42 per cent area in Pakistan, whilst the dry region of India has the same total area affected as Pakistan (11 million hectares). Salinity and water-logging are the other major concerns of land degradation in the irrigated command areas and in the coastal regions. India, Bangladesh and Pakistan together have 14.23 million hectares salt-affected area. Thus, arable land is becoming scarce for many South Asian countries. There are growing land inequalities in South Asian countries. In Nepal, for instance, five per cent households own about 37 per cent arable land while 47 per cent households own only 15 per cent of the total arable land (UNDP 2004).

Among these challenges, this chapter focuses on COVID-19 impacts on air pollution and climate change, and its implications for South Asian environmental security. Air pollution and climate change have been purposively chosen.

COVID-19 and Environment in South Asia

The COVID-19 pandemic has abundantly shown to the world that human actions can make a difference when it concerns the environment and environmental security. Since the beginning of the global spread of

COVID-19, the world has been witnessing a qualitative change in environmental conditions from local to global levels. As indicated above, South Asia is one of the dangerously polluted regions in the world. The areas of environmental degradation in the region are manifold and multidimensional. A few of these aspects, such as air pollution and global warming, have been positively influenced by the COVID-19 pandemic. Besides, the COVID-19 pandemic has placed a restraint on unfettered consumption patterns and inspired cleanliness at different levels—from family to office. This section has specifically focused impacts of COVID-19 on air pollution and climate change.

Air Pollution

Several studies show that there are clear linkages between air pollution and COVID-19. On the one hand, air pollution leads to the increasing vulnerability of COVID-19 (Setti et al. 2020; Tian et al. 2020). It is found that people with long-term exposure to air pollution are mostly vulnerable to COVID-19. On the other hand, due to the outbreak of COVID-19 and its consequent measures, i.e., lockdown measures have had a positive impact on air quality (McGrath, March 19, 2020). As we have seen, to contain the COVID-19 global pandemic, there are lockdown measures and business closures, cancellation of flights and other journeys globally and regionally that have contributed to a substantial reduction of nitrogen dioxide, a serious air pollutant, which has resulted in improved air quality globally. For instance, the measures taken to control COVID-19 have improved air quality in Europe substantially (European Environment Agency, March 25, 2020). It is noted that just after two weeks of lockdown in UK, nitrogen dioxide pollution was reduced by 60 per cent in some cities compared to the same period in 2019 (Monks 2020). According to NASA, NO pollution in New York and other major metropolitan areas in north-eastern USA was 30 per cent lower in March 2020, compared to the monthly average from 2015 to 2019 (cited in Monks 2020). Lauri Myllyvirta (April 30, 2020) writes that in April, 2020 alone, due to coronavirus measures, there was a 40 per cent reduction of nitrogen dioxide (NO_2) pollution and 10 per cent reduction in the average level of particulate matter pollution which resulted in 11,000 avoided deaths from air pollution in Europe alone. China emits about 50 per cent of NO_2 emissions in Asia. Notably, the country emitted 40 mega tonnes of nitrogen oxide in 2019. Due to the lockdown measures, over half a billion people across China were in lockdown, which reduced the use of cars significantly. It is noted that 'the 40 per cent drop in NO at 2019 levels for January and February in some areas equates to removing a whopping 192,000 cars' off the road and this reducing NO_2 emission (Monks 2020).

Lockdown measures have also contributed to the reduction of air pollution significantly in South Asia. Dhaka, the capital city of Bangladesh, often hits the headlines by becoming one of the worst air polluted cities in the world. But due to the novel coronavirus, the measures taken by Bangladesh have improved air quality 'significantly' (*UNB News*, May 22, 2020; *New Age*, April 15, 2020).

It is claimed that transport, industries, power plants, construction activities, biomass and refuse burning, road dust re-suspension and residential activities, restaurants, landfill fires are primarily responsible for air pollution in India (Central Pollution Control Board, March 31, 2020) as well as in other South Asian nations. Just after one week of lockdown in India, the Central Pollution Control Board (March 31, 2020) found a substantial improvement of air quality in India. According to scientists, due to the reduction of industrial and human activities, air quality, water quality, biodiversity has improved in India. In addition, noise pollution has also been reduced in India (*The Hindu*, June 4, 2020). James Poetzscher writes in *The Hindu* that 'India's nationwide lockdown, in particular, has had stunning effects on air pollution levels. With citizens quarantined at home, road transportation and power plant operations have come to a grinding halt, and pollution levels across the country, especially in typically smoggy cities, have fallen to dramatic lows' (Poetzscher 2020).

Air quality has also improved in Pakistan due to coronavirus impacts. In this regard, Farzana Altaf Shah, Director General of Pakistan Environment Protection Agency, contends that 'We have seen good quality air days before, but you can feel the fresher breath of air more than ever in Islamabad. It only goes to show the major impact human activities have on the climate of our city. This brief period of cleaner air should send a message for people to push for long-term changes' (quoted in Shahid 2020). COVID-19 has also impacted community mobility significantly (Table 2), which has contributed to the reduction of fossil fuel use, thus improving air quality.

Table 2: COVID-19 Community Mobility in South Asia (Percentage change from baseline as of May 9, 2020)

Country	Retail & recreation	Grocery & pharmacy	Parks	Transit stations	Workplaces	Residential
Afghanistan	–40	–17	–20	–41	–30	+12
Bangladesh	–64	–42	–33	–59	–34	+20
Bhutan	-	-	-	-	-	-
India	–80	–32	–62	–57	–49	+25
Maldives	-	-	-	-	-	-
Nepal	–67	–52	–44	–58	–35	+17
Pakistan	–52	–34	–32	–45	–30	+16
Sri Lanka	–82	–80	–54	–76	–49	+33

Source: https://www.google.com/covid19/mobility/

Table 2 demonstrates that a large number of people are staying at home except for limited movement during lockdown days in South Asia, which impacted on the use of ground traffic. In India and Sri Lanka, for instance, there was a 49 per cent drop in the number of people reporting for work while it was a 30 to 35 per cent drop for other South Asian countries. There is also a significant drop in other sectors, i.e., retail and recreation, which impacted the improvement of air quality in South Asia.

Climate Change

While the whole world is concerned mostly on the impacts of COVID-19 on health and economy, it becomes pertinent to investigate its implications on global climate change as it impacts everyone on a larger scale. Thus it becomes essential to investigate: To what extent does COVID-19 impact global climate change? Matt McGrath reports in *BBC News* (May 6, 2020) that 'No war, no recession, no previous pandemic has had such a dramatic impact on emissions of CO_2 over the past century as COVID-19 has in a few short months'. The Second World War had a significant impact as carbon emissions fell globally, a drop of around 800 million tonnes. Due to the global recession in the early 1980s and the oil crisis of the late 1970s, CO_2 emissions fell by approximately one billion tonnes. The world also witnessed 450 million tonnes of CO_2 drop during the 2008-2009 Global Financial Crisis. In 2009, there was minus 1.4 per cent decline of CO_2 emissions. It is believed that the COVID-19 global pandemic will surpass earlier records. Le Quere et al. (2020), in their study, find that due to the worldwide lockdown measures, global carbon emissions declined by 17 per cent as on 7 April 2020 relative to the mean level of emissions in 2019 (Table 3).

Table 3: Global Carbon Emission Decline for Each Sector on the Day with the Maximum Change (7 April 2020)

Sector	Daily carbon emission decline (7 April 2020)
Power	−7.4
Industry	−19
Surface transport	−36
Public	−21
Residential	+2.8
Aviation	−60
Total	−17

Source: Le Quere et al. (2020).

Table 3 demonstrates that 60 per cent carbon emission declined in the aviation sector alone, while 36 per cent diminished in the surface transport sector. Only in the residential sector, there is an increase in carbon emission by 2.8 per cent. However, global carbon emission declined by 17 per cent on April 7, 2020 due to worldwide lockdown measures. Until the end of April 2020, it is estimated that global carbon emission had dropped by 1,048 million tonnes equivalent to a minus 8.6 per cent decrease over January–April 2019 (Le Quere et al. 2020). In China, CO_2 emission declined by 242 million tonnes and in the USA by 207 million tonnes. Europe holds the third position with a drop of 123 million tonnes, while India holds the fourth position with a fall of 98 million tonnes (Le Quere et al. 2020).

According to the International Energy Agency (IEA), due to COVID-19 impacts, the demand for energy declined globally by 3.8 per cent in the first quarter of 2020, mainly felt in March 2020 when Asia, Europe, North America experienced lockdown measures (IEA 2020). The world will use 6 per cent less energy in 2020, which will contribute to the fall of carbon emissions significantly. More specifically, IEA notes that there will be a nine per cent drop in oil demand, while coal use could decline by eight per cent in 2020 due to the coronavirus outbreak. The use/demand of gas and nuclear power will also fall. IEA (2020) also claims that

> Global CO_2 emissions are expected to decline by 8%, or almost 2.6 gigatonnes (Gt), to levels of 10 years ago. Such a year-on-year reduction would be the largest ever, six times larger than the previous record reduction of 0.4 Gt in 2009—caused by the global financial crisis—and twice as large as the combined total of all previous reductions since the end of World War II. As after previous crises, however, the rebound in emissions may be larger than the decline, unless the wave of investment to restart the economy is dedicated to cleaner and more resilient energy infrastructure.

There are also negative implications of COVID-19 on climate change. It disrupts the global environmental negotiations, including the conference of parties (COP) which might delay/impede the legally binding agreement to cut carbon emissions. COP 26 international climate summit has been postponed until 2021. Thus the world's largest emitters, including China and the USA might utilise the absence of any legally binding agreement to accelerate their economic growth and thus increase the volume of carbon emissions.

Since South Asian states maintained lockdown and shutdown measures to contain the spread of the novel coronavirus, it contributed to the decline of carbon emissions. However, as South Asian states (except India) contribute less to the volume of global carbon emissions, the declining amount of carbon emission is also minimal. For the first time in four decades, carbon emission was declined in India. In March 2020, there was a 15 per cent decline of carbon emission while it declined by 30 per cent in April 2020 (Myllyvirta and Dahiya 2020).

The COVID-19 pandemic has made a positive impact on the consumption patterns of people in South Asia. As a growing economy with rising numbers of middle-class people and millionaires, the region has developed unplanned and unsustainable consumption patterns, which have an enormous impact on the environment through air pollution, resource crisis, global warming, food adulteration and health hazards. Many reports reveal that South Asians are consuming adulterated and substandard food everyday that increases the risks of malnutrition, food poisoning and fatal diseases like cancer. According to a report published in the *Dhaka Tribune* (February 5, 2020), in Bangladesh more than 4.5 million people are at health risk for consuming adulterated and contaminated food every day. With the reduction of demand for food during the pandemic, people are less prone to health hazards caused by adulterated food. People have also got an opportunity to reflect on their destructive consumption patterns that play a role to germinate greed in the minds of corrupt producers and traders. The pandemic virus has also inspired people to maintain cleanliness in society. South Asia has a poor record of cleanliness for which environmental degradation gets further worsened every day. COVID-19 has taught a lesson to the people of South Asia that cleanliness not only fights environmental degradation but also maintains human health.

Implications for South Asian Environmental Security

As mentioned earlier, air pollution and climate change have been purposively chosen to understand the impacts of COVID-19 on South Asian environmental security. Here, how air pollution and climate change become sources of insecurity for the South Asian people will be investigated. Air pollution contributes to deaths. According to the WHO, 'An estimated 4.2 million premature deaths globally are linked to ambient air pollution, mainly from heart disease, stroke, chronic obstructive pulmonary disease, lung cancer, and acute respiratory infections in children' (WHO, n.d.). Additionally, two United States-based institutes—the Health Effects Institute (HEI) and Institute for Health Metrics and Evaluation (IHME)—in their study titled, 'State of Global Air-2019', find that in 2017 alone at least 123, 000 people died in Bangladesh, 1.2 million people died in India, and 128,000 died in Pakistan due to indoor and outdoor air pollution (*Dhaka Tribune*, April 4, 2019; Ashok, April 3, 2019). The Centre for Science and Environment (CSE), in its report titled *State of India's Environment*, mentions that 'Air pollution is responsible for 12.5 per cent of all deaths in India. Its impact on children is equally worrying. Over 100,000 children below the age of five die due to bad air in the country' (*The Indian Express*, June 5, 2019). The number of premature deaths in 2018 was 1,000,000 in India while it was 96,000 in Bangladesh due to air pollution (generated by burning fossil fuel) related diseases (Farrow et al. 2020).

The headline of *Al Jazeera* (January 16, 2019), i.e., 'Kabul's air pollution kills more people than war' underscores the severity of air pollution as a source of insecurity for the Afghan people. According to the Ministry of Health, Afghanistan, air pollution causes more than 3,000 deaths in the country where mostly children are vulnerable (*Al Jazeera*, January 16, 2019). In one week in December 2019, more than 17 people died in Kabul due to air-pollution related diseases, particularly respiratory diseases ((*Al Jazeera*, December 31, 2019). According to a 2005-2006 United Nations Environment Programme (UNEP) report, 60 per cent of the people in Kabul are exposed to a high level of air pollution containing particular matter, nitrous oxides and sulphur oxides. The Afghan Ministry of Health notes that there were around 480,000 reported cases of respiratory illness and asthma between 2002 and 2010 (cited in Goudsouzian 2011). This illness could be prevented if environmental regulations were implemented strictly. Additionally, UNEP notes that international standards are not maintained in using most of the fuels in Afghanistan, which contain high levels of lead. The Afghan Ministry of Health conducted a study in 2009 where it found that the blood samples of 80 per cent of some 200 Kabul residents contained lead. Atiq Sediqi, an Environmental Management Systems Auditor, and an adviser to the Afghan Ministry of Mines, contends that 'It is the lead in the environment that poisons the brains of Afghan children living in urban sprawls and reduces their learning ability and other air pollutants that are threatening the public health every day, killing many citizens every day' (cited in Goudsouzian 2011).

For other South Asian countries, though the number of deaths is less compared to Bangladesh, India and Pakistan, people's health in general and children's health, in particular, is badly affected. Air pollution also leads to adverse pregnancy outcomes. The WHO notes that 'Maternal exposure to ambient air pollution is associated with adverse birth outcomes, such as low birth weight, pre-term birth and small gestational age births. Emerging evidence also suggests that ambient air pollution may affect diabetes and neurological development in children' (WHO, n.d.). Thus, air pollution bears threats to a healthy and productive life for South Asian people, which can be defined as environmental insecurity.

As mentioned in earlier sections, air quality in South Asia has improved significantly due to COVID-19, which has a positive impact on people's health, especially on that of children. The picture is similar for other South Asian countries. Thus, COVID-19 has been imperative for improvement of people's lives and improve environmental security in the context of air pollution. Tens of thousands of premature deaths in South Asia can be avoided if air pollution is controlled.

With regard to the impacts of climate change, one can mention that South Asia has faced an increased number of natural disasters due to the impact of global warming and climate change. This has caused tens of thousands of deaths, as shown earlier. These deaths could also have been avoided if the reduction of carbon emissions could be continued as was in the COVID-19 period. In addition, the negative impacts of climate change will lead to the rise of environmental refugees in South Asia and beyond. Although 'the projections vary from as few as 50 million to as many as 500 million, the problem is clear: Millions of people around the world will be displaced because of rising sea levels, desertification, drought, weather-related flooding, and other environmental changes' (Vaughn 2011: 331). There is likely to be intra-state and inter-state tensions due to these environmental refugees in South Asia and beyond which has clear environmental security implications.

The COVID-19 global pandemic has raised cognitive awareness towards the environment, which needs to be nurtured for the long-term interest of the region and beyond. COVID-19 has been imperative for South Asian environmental security in the context of air pollution and climate change. As discussed above, air pollution and climate change have been significant sources of environmental insecurity for millions of people in South Asia. The improvement of air quality and the reduction of greenhouse emissions brought short term positive impacts in the context of environmental security in South Asia. For long term positive implications, South Asian states need to seriously consider the following policy imperatives.

Policy Imperatives

Focusing on Environmentally Sensitive Climate Policy

In the long term, the world needs to focus on climate policy that encourages the deployment of clean technologies and reductions in demand for fossil fuels. The policy needs to work for the planet instead of the economic interests of the corporate world. In this context, visionary global leadership becomes essential to reach net-zero carbon emissions. It would be wiser to take a lesson from the COVID-19 global pandemic and build a sustainable future based on a climate policy that puts the environment ahead of the economy or maintains a balance between them. Pascal Peduzzi, Director of UNEP/GRID-Geneva, contends that 'COVID-19 provides us a chance to take stock of the risks we are taking in our unsustainable relationship with our environment and seize the opportunity to rebuild our economies in a more environmentally responsible way' (quoted in UN Environment Programme, May 11, 2020). At the same time, it would be suicidal to focus on recovering the economic loss from the lockdown measures and thus increase the use of fossil fuels. This will, in fact, increase carbon emissions, which will ultimately destroy the planet. Constructive societal response is also necessary to reduce carbon emissions.

Promoting Renewable Energy and other Low-carbon Sources

Lockdown measures are not a permanent solution to air pollution or climate change. Instead, the use of renewable energy and low-carbon sources needs to be promoted. It is argued that the improvements of air quality or decline of global carbon emissions during the lockdown days regionally and globally could be permanent if the use of fossil fuels could be replaced by the use of renewable energy and other low-carbon uses (Monks 2020). The *Himal South Asian* in its editorial (April 22, 2020) notes that 'The current moment [COVID-19] presents an opportunity for governments in South Asia to rethink their energy priorities and explore investments in more sustainable and renewable energy sources'. Ironically, the use of coal for energy production has been rampant for many South Asian countries, especially India (Takahashi 2001). Burning coal causes trans-boundary air pollution. Thus, the use of coal power plants in South Asia needs to be discouraged by governments and corporations. Instead of profit-maximising activities, the welfare and well-being of the people in South Asia need to be taken into consideration by the business community. Róisín Commane, a professor from Columbia University in New York, contends that 'personal behaviour really isn't going to fix the carbon emission problem. We need a systematic change in how energy is generated and transmitted' (quoted in McGrath 2020b). Consequently, renewable energy in the ocean sources needs to be utilised. More specifically, solar and wind power needs to be encouraged. In fact, to sustain a habitable world for humans and other species, there is no alternative to focus on renewable energy and low carbon sources.

Mainstreaming Air Pollution

COVID-19 has shown that air pollution in South Asia can be controlled. Thus air pollution needs to be mainstreamed in both policy and academic discourse in South Asia. In 2014, China declared war on pollution. Consequently, China reduced emissions and prohibited new coal-fired power plants in the most polluted regions, including Beijing. The country also shut down coal mines. Instead of coal, it [China] focused on natural gas, restricted the number of cars in large cities, including Beijing and Shanghai. As a result, China succeeded in reducing pollution significantly. It is argued that if China continues its emission reductions, 'residents will see significant improvements to their health, extending their life spans by months or years' (Greenstone 2018). In the case of South Asia, as mentioned earlier, the neo-liberal economic model, the principle of profit-over-people is followed. And thus, economic growth gets prioritised over environmental protection. In this scenario, South Asian countries need to declare war on air pollution and cut pollution significantly for the well-being of their people. Instead of deforestation, South Asian states need to focus on tree plantation. Public health policy needs to be prioritised to face the upcoming public health disaster due to air pollution.

Reinforcing Regional Initiatives

U.C. Jha (2004:1669) writes that 'The problem of environmental degradation in south Asia is partly due to political mistrust in the region'. Despite such a claim, it is observed that South Asian states embraced some regional initiatives to promote regional cooperation on the environment. For instance, in 1982, South Asian countries formed the South Asia Co-operative Environment Programme (SACEP) to deepen regional cooperation on the environment. SACEP became a milestone in the regional cooperation process on the environment. In addition, South Asian countries also formed the South Asian Association for Regional Cooperation (SAARC) in 1985 to promote regional cooperation. Both SACEP and SAARC have pursued regional cooperation on the environment. In 1987, SAARC adopted its Environment Action Plan. In 1998, under the purview of SACEP, South Asian countries adopted the Malé Declaration on control and prevention of air pollution and its likely trans-boundary effects for South Asia. According to SACEP, 'The declaration emphasises the need for countries to carry forward, or initiate, studies and programmes on air pollution in each country of South Asia' (SACEP n.d.). Notably, SACEP implemented an Action Plan called Strategy and Programme in the format of different phases. Key areas of activity included capacity building and awareness-raising; systematic information exchange and intra-regional technology transfer; training on environmental management and institutional development, promotion of policy measures to control emissions of air pollution and the assurance of sustainability in the region. In 2004, SACEP and SAARC signed a MoU on cooperation for the protection of the environment of the region. At the Thirteenth Summit meeting of SAARC held in Dhaka on 12-13 November 2005 South Asian states adopted the Dhaka Declaration on South Asia's

Environmental Challenges and Natural Disasters where they emphasised the promotion of regional cooperation on environmental issues, i.e., natural disasters. They also decided to consider the modalities for having a Regional Environment Treaty in furthering environmental cooperation among the SAARC Member-States. Thus, regional initiatives already exist but need to be reinforced for the enhancement of South Asian environmental security.

Ending North-South Divide in Global Environmental Politics and Reducing Emissions

South Asia alone cannot solve the problem of climate change. Climate change is a global issue, which requires a global solution. And in the process of a global solution, the north-south divide in global environmental politics has remained an impediment. In addition, the withdrawal of the USA (a major polluter) from the Paris climate agreement provides a negative message for global environmental security. Other major polluters might be motivated not to comply with the global environmental agreements, which will be counterproductive for the entire global environment. Emissions from burning fossil fuels need to be reduced significantly. In this case, new technologies that contribute to emission reduction need to be introduced and promoted. It is argued that 'Reducing emissions is a wise long term investment that contributes to several development goals and ultimately will yield substantial benefits' (UNECE n.d.). An emission limit needs to be strictly followed globally to confront climate change and thus save the planet from destruction. In this case, there is no alternative but cooperation to face life-threatening climate change. The states in the world need to come out from realist or neo-realist paradigm to define national interest and need to remove all the divisions whether North-South or South-South in global environmental politics to save humanity from environmental insecurity.

Conclusion

The chapter has investigated the implications of COVID-19 on South Asian environmental security with particular reference to air pollution and climate change. It finds that environmental insecurity from air pollution and climate change has been a grave concern for millions of people in South Asia. The COVID-19 global pandemic brought not only challenges but also opportunities. The global environment is recovering due to the lockdown measures and business closures against the outbreak of COVID-19. COVID-19 put a pause on the way people were destroying the global environment. The impacts of COVID-19 in the context of air pollution and climate change, i.e., the improvement of air quality and the reduction of carbon emissions has been imperative for the enhancement of environmental security in the South Asian region and beyond.

Air pollution and climate change affect everyone, whether poor or rich, powerless or powerful. For a bright and sustainable future for South Asian states, there is no alternative but to ensure a safe, healthy environment, which requires regional and global cooperation. As Myers (1989:23) contends, 'The world is increasingly interdependent environmentally as well as economically. Pollution, whether air- or water-borne, is readily transported from one country to another'. Thus, all the stakeholders concerned, both state and non-state actors, need to come forward to address the menace of air pollution and climate change in South Asia and beyond. As argued earlier, regional cooperation initiatives need to be reinforced to protect the South Asian environment and thus ensure environmental security. In addition, to save the environment, individual interests need to be replaced by the common interest of people in the region. In the context of Afghanistan, for instance, Saba notes that 'Individual interests prevent them [political leaders] from seriously implementing regulations. They think of immediate economic gains, rather than the long-term environmental damages' (cited in Goudsouzian 2011). This chapter concludes by saying that for the betterment and well-being of the people of the region, there is no alternative but to enhance environmental security. This requires addressing both air pollution and climate change, which need to be prioritised in the policymaking and execution for the collective future of South Asia.

REFERENCES

ADB (2013, March 6). Clean technologies could cut South Asia emissions by a fifth by 2020 at little cost. News Release. Retrieved from https://www.adb.org/news/clean-technologies-could-cut-south-asia-emissions-fifth-2020-little-cost

Adlakha, N. (2020, February 28). No country for climate refugees. *The Hindu*. Retrieved from https://www.thehindu.com/opinion/columns/how-the-climate-crisis-is-uprooting-more-people-than-war/article30942108.ece

Ahmed, M. and S. Suphachalasai. (2014). *Assessing the costs of climate change and adaptation in South Asia*. Mandaluyong City, Philippines: Asian Development Bank.

Allenby, B. R. (2000). Environmental security: Concept and implementation. *International Political Science Review*, 21 (1), 5–21.

Al Jazeera (2019, January 16). Kabul's air pollution kills more people than war. Retrieved from https://www.aljazeera.com/news/2019/01/kabuls-air-pollution-kills-people-war-190116094807604.html

Al Jazeera (2019, December 31). Kabul: 17 killed due to hazardous levels of air pollution. Retrieved from https://www.aljazeera.com/news/2019/12/kabul-17-killed-due-hazardous-levels-air-pollution-191231062957367.html

Al Jazeera (2020, January 21). Davos: World needs to prepare for 'millions' of climate refugees. Retrieved from https://www.aljazeera.com/ajimpact/davos-world-prepare-millions-climate-refugees-200121175217520.html

Amin, M. A. (2018, December 17). Reckless plastic waste dumping greatly endangering Bay of Bengal. *Dhaka Tribune*. Retrieved from https://www.dhakatribune.com/bangladesh/environment/2018/12/17/reckless-plastic-waste-dumping-greatly-endangering-bay-of-bengal

Ashok, S. (2019, April 3). Air pollution killed 1.2 million people in India in 2017, says report; bigger killer than smoking. *The Indian Express*. Retrieved from https://indianexpress.com/article/india/air-pollution-killed-1-2-million-people-in-india-in-2017-says-report-bigger-killer-than-smoking-5655861/

Azad, A.K. (2011). Preface. In D. Sarkar, A.K. Azad, S.K. Singh & N. Akter (eds.), *Strategies for arresting land degradation in South Asian countries* (pp. viii-ix). Dhaka: SAARC Agriculture Centre.

Barnett, J., Matthew, R.A. & O'Brien, K. L. (2010). Global Environmental Change and Human Security: An Introduction. In R. A. Matthew, J. Barnett, B. McDonald, and K. L. O'Brien (Eds.), *Global environmental change and human security* (3-32), Boston: MIT Press.

BBC News (2018, June 2). Whale that died off Thailand had eaten 80 plastic bags. Retrieved from https://www.bbc.com/news/world-asia-44344468

BBC News (2020, April 29). Coronavirus: Wild animals enjoy freedom of a quieter world. Retrieved from https://www.bbc.com/news/world-52459487

Booth, K. (1991). Security and emancipation. *Review of International Studies*, 17 (4) 313-326.

Buzan, Barry. 1983. *People, States and Fear: National Security Problem in International Relations*. (2nd Edition), Sussex: Wheatsheaf Books Ltd.

Central Pollution Control Board.(2020, March 31). Impact of janta curfew & lockdown on air quality. Ministry of Environment, Forest and Climate Change, Govt. of India, Delhi.

Chandrasekaran, M. (2019, August 9). Poor air quality affects everyone's wellbeing, but children are worst affected. *Firstpost*. Retrieved from https://www.firstpost.com/health/poor-air-quality-affects-everyones-wellbeing-but-children-are-worst-affected 7135131.html

Chatterjee, P. (2015, April 2). Leave Delhi: That's what doctors are prescribing to patients with serious respiratory ailments. *The Indian Express*. Retrieved from https://indianexpress.com/article/india/india-others/leave-delhi/

Dhaka Tribune (2019, April 3). Children in South Asia hardest hit by air pollution. Retrieved from https://www.dhakatribune.com/world/south-asia/2019/04/03/children-in-south-asia-hardest-hit-by-air-pollution

Dhaka Tribune (2019, April 4). Report: Air pollution killed 123,000 people in Bangladesh in 2017. Retrieved from https://www.dhakatribune.com/bangladesh/nation/2019/04/04/report-air-pollution-killed-123-000-people-in-bangladesh-in-2017

Dhaka Tribune (2020 February 5), The high cost of consuming adulterated food.

European Environment Agency (2020, March 25). Air pollution goes down as Europe takes hard measures to combat coronavirus. Retrieved from https://www.eea.europa.eu/highlights/air-pollution-goes-down-as

Fallesen, D., Khan, H., Tehsin, A. & Abbhi, A. (2019, November 11). South Asia needs to act as one to fight climate change. World Bank Blogs. Retrieved from https://blogs.worldbank.org/endpovertyinsouthasia/south-asia-needs-act-one-fight-climate-change

Farrow, A., Miller, K.A. & Myllyvirta, L. (2020, February). Toxic air: The price of fossil fuels. Seoul: Greenpeace Southeast Asia. 44 pp. February 2020.

Goudsouzian, T. (2011, March 17). Something in the air in Kabul. *Al Jazeera*. Retrieved from https://www.aljazeera.com/indepth/features/2011/03/201131514261904290.html

Greenstone, M. (2018, March 12). Four years after declaring war on pollution, China is winning. *The New York Times*. Retrieved from https://www.nytimes.com/2018/03/12/upshot/china-pollution-environment-longer-lives.html

Hamilton, C., Bonneuil, C.& Gemenne, F. (Eds.) (2015). *The Anthropocene and the global environmental crisis: Rethinking modernity in a new epoch*. Abingdon, Oxon: Routledge.

Harrabin, R. (2017, December 5). Ocean plastic a 'planetary crisis' – UN. *BBC News*. Retrieved from https://www.bbc.com/news/science-environment-42225915

Himal South Asian (2020, April 22). Why South Asia's air is cleaner this Earth Day. Retrieved from https://www.himalmag.com/why-southasias-air-is-cleaner-this-earth-day/

Hossain, S. (2020, March 30, 2020). Kuakata's red crabs return to the beach. *The Daily Star*. Retrieved from https://www.thedailystar.net/online/news/kuakatas-red-crabs-return-the-beach-1887712

Homer-Dixon, T. F. (1991). On the threshold: Environmental changes and causes of acute conflict. *International Security*, 16 (2), 76-116.

Homer-Dixon, T. F. (1994). Environmental scarcities and violent conflict: Evidence from cases. *International Security*, 19 (1), 5-40.

Hough, P. (2019). Back to the future: environmental security in nineteenth century global politics. *Global Security: Health, Science and Policy*, 4 (1), 1-13, DOI: 10.1080/23779497.2019.1663128

Islam, M. M. M. (2019, August 10). Alarming plastic pollution in the Bay of Bengal. *The Daily Star.* Retrieved from https://www.thedailystar.net/opinion/environment/news/alarming-plastic-pollution-the-bay-bengal-1784278

IEA (2020, April). Global energy review 2020. Retrieved from https://www.iea.org/reports/global-energy-review-2020

Jha, U. C. (2004). Environmental issues and SAARC. *Economic and Political Weekly,* 39 (17), 1666-1671.

Le Quéré, C., Jackson, R. B., Jones, M. W., Smith, A. J. P., Abernethy, S., Andrew, R. M., De-Gol, A. J., Willis, D. R., Shan, Y., Canadell, J. G., Friedlingstein, P., Creutzig, F.& Peters, G. P. (2020). Temporary reduction in daily global CO_2 emissions during the COVID-19 forced confinement. *Nature Climate Change.* https://doi.org/10.1038/s41558-020-0797-x

Lipu, T. I. (2020, April 3). As humans away, other creatures stage comeback. *The Independent.* Retrieved from http://www.theindependentbd.com/post/243451

Marsh, S. (2020, January 8). On the frontline of the climate emergency, Bangladesh adapts. *The Guardian.* Retrieved from https://www.theguardian.com/world/2020/jan/08/on-the-frontline-of-the-climate-emergency-bangladesh-adapts

Matthew, R. A., Barnett, J., Bryan McDonald, B., and Karen L. O'Brien, K. L. (eds.) (2010). *Global environmental change and human security.* Boston: MIT Press.

Mathews, J. T. (1989). Redefining security. *Foreign Affairs.* 68 (2), 162-177

McGrath, M. (2020a, March 19). Coronavirus: Air pollution and CO_2 fall rapidly as virus spreads. *BBC News.* Retrieved from https://www.bbc.com/news/science-environment-51944780

McGrath, M. (2020b, May 6). Climate change and coronavirus: Five charts about the biggest carbon crash. *BBC News.* Retrieved from https://www.bbc.com/news/science-environment-52485712

Molla, M. A. (2019, March 6). Living in toxic air. *The Daily Star.* Retrieved from https://www.thedailystar.net/frontpage/dhaka-second-most-polluted-air-city-in-world-living-toxic-air-1711213

Monks, P. (2020, April 15). Coronavirus: lockdown's effect on air pollution provides rare glimpse of low-carbon future. *The Conversation.* Retrieved from https://theconversation.com/coronavirus-lockdowns-effect-on-air-pollution-provides-rare-glimpse-of-low-carbon-future-134685

Myllyvirta, L. (2020, April 30). 11,000 air pollution-related deaths avoided in Europe as coal, oil consumption plummet. Centre for Research on Energy and Clean Air. Retrieved from https://energyandcleanair.org/air-pollution-deaths-avoided-in-europe-as-coal-oil-plummet/

Myllyvirta, L. & Dahiya, S. (2020, May 12). Analysis: India's CO_2 emissions fall for first time in four decades amid coronavirus. Carbon Brief. Retrieved from https://www.carbonbrief.org/analysis-indias-co2-emissions-fall-for-first-time-in-four-decades-amid-coronavirus

Myers, N. (1989, Spring). Environment and security. *Foreign Policy,* 74, 23-41.

New Age. (2020, April 15). Dhaka air quality slightly improves amid lockdown. Retrieved from https://www.newagebd.net/article/104433/dhaka-air-quality-slightly-improves-amid-lockdown

Ney, S. (1999). Environmental security: A critical overview. *Innovation: The European Journal of Social Science Research,* 12(1), 7-30, DOI: 10.1080/13511610.1999.9968585

Ngumbi, E. (2020, January 3). Putting a price on soil. *Project Syndicate*. Retrieved from https://www.project-syndicate.org/commentary/soil-agriculture-erosion-climate-regenerative-nitrogen-fertilizers-overgrazing-deforestation-by-esther-ngumbi-2020-01?barrier=accesspaylog

Pennington, J. (2016, October 27). Every minute, one garbage truck of plastic is dumped into our oceans. This has to stop. World Economic Forum. Retrieved from https://www.weforum.org/agenda/2016/10/every-minute-one-garbage-truck-of-plastic-is-dumped-into-our-oceans/

Poetzscher, J. (2020, May 12). The effect of COVID-19 on India's air quality. *The Hindu*. Retrieved from https://www.thehindubusinessline.com/opinion/columns/the-effect-of-COVID-19-on-indias-air-quality/article31564038.ece

Saferworld (2008). *Human security in Bangladesh*. Retrieved from https://www.saferworld.org.uk/resources/publications/323-human-security-in-bangladesh

Schupska, S. (2015, February 12). New science paper calculates magnitude of plastic waste going into the ocean. Retrieved from https://news.uga.edu/new-science-paper-magnitude-plastic-waste-going-into-ocean-0215/

Setti, L., Passarini, F., Gennaro, G. D., Baribieri, P., Perrone, M. G., Borelli, M., Palmisani, J., Gilio, A. D., Torboli, V., Pallavicini, A., Ruscio, M., Piscitelli, P. & Miani, A. (2020). SARS-Cov-2 RNA Found on Particulate Matter of Bergamo in Northern Italy: First Preliminary Evidence. *medRxiv*.doi: https://doi.org/10.1101/2020.04.15.20065995

Shahid, J. (2020, April 3). Lockdown improves quality of air over capital. *Dawn*. Retrieved from https://www.dawn.com/news/1545988

Singh, A. K. & Singh, S. K. (2011). Keynote paper on strategies for arresting land degradation in South Asian countries. In D. Sarkar, A. K. Azad, S.K. Singh & N. Akter (eds.), *Strategies for arresting land degradation in South Asian countries* (pp.1-31). Dhaka: SAARC Agriculture Centre.

Sky News (2017, December 12). Just 10 rivers carry 90% of plastic polluting the oceans. Retrieved from https://news.sky.com/story/just-10-rivers-carry-90-of-plastic-polluting-the-oceans-11167581

The Daily Star (2018, April 24). Resilient infrastructure: For the blue economy. Retrieved from https://www.thedailystar.net/round-tables/the-blue-economy-1566883

The Daily Star (2019, December 12). Rise in sea level may reduce 24pc cropland by 2045. Retrieved from https://www.thedailystar.net/business/news/rise-sea-level-may-reduce-24pc-cropland-2045-1839160

The Daily Star (2020, January 15). Around 4cr people might be displaced due to climate change in Bangladesh: PM. Retrieved from ohttps://www.thedailystar.net/country/climate-change-in-bangladesh-around-4-crore-people-might-be-displaced-1854463

The Hindu (2020, June 4). COVID-19 lockdown-like interventions may help combat air pollution in India, say scientists. Retrieved from https://www.thehindu.com/sci-tech/energy-and-environment/COVID-19-lockdown-like-interventions-may-help-combat-air-pollution-in-india-say-scientists/article31746151.ece

The Japan Times, (2020, April 18). With fishing fleets tied up due to COVID-19, marine life has a chance to recover. Retrieved from https://www.japantimes.co.jp/news/2020/04/18/world/science-health-world/fishing-coronavirus-marine-life/#.XsV29qZS_IU

The Indian Express (2019, May 23). Air pollution may up childhood anxiety, depression, finds study. Retrieved from https://indianexpress.com/article/lifestyle/health/air-pollution-may-up-childhood-anxiety-depression-study-5743740/

The Indian Express (2019, June 5). 1 lakh kids under 5 years of age die due to air pollution each year: Study. Retrieved from https://indianexpress.com/article/lifestyle/health/1-lakh-kids-under-5-years-of-age-die-due-to-air-pollution-each-year-study-5766833/

The Indian Express (2019, July 10). Air pollution may age your lungs faster, says study. Retrieved from https://indianexpress.com/article/lifestyle/health/air-pollution-may-age-your-lungs-faster-study-5823344/

Times of India (2020, March 24). Videos of dolphin playing in Mumbai sea amid COVID-19 lockdown are going viral. Retrieved from https://timesofindia.indiatimes.com/travel/destinations/videos-of-dolphin-playing-in-mumbai-sea-amid-COVID-19-lockdown-are-going-viral/as74787988.cms

Tian, H., Liu, Y., Song, H., Wu, C., Li, B., Kraemer, M. U. G., Zheng, P., Yan, X., Jia, G., Zheng, Y., Stenseth, N. C. & Dye, C. (2020, April 24). Risk of COVID-19 is associated with long-term exposure to air pollution. *medRxiv*. preprintdoi: https://doi.org/10.1101/2020.04.21.20073700

UN Sustainable Development Goals Blog. (2017, December 6). Millions of babies, mostly in South Asia, risk brain damage from breathing toxic air, UNICEF warns. Retrieved from https://www.un.org/sustainabledevelopment/blog/2017/12/millions-babies-mostly-south-asia-risk-brain-damage-breathing-toxic-air-unicef-warns/

UNB News (2020, May 22). Dhaka's air quality improves significantly. Retrieved from https://unb.com.bd/category/Bangladesh/dhakas-air-quality-improves-significantly/51966

UNDP (1994). *Human development report 1994*. New York: Oxford University Press.

UNDP (2004). *Nepal human development report: Empowerment and poverty reduction*. Kathmandu: United Nations Development Programme.

UNECE (n.d.). Air pollution and economic development. Retrieved from https://www.unece.org/environmental-policy/conventions/envlrtapwelcome/cross-sectoral-linkages/air-pollution-and-economic-development.html

UN Environment Programme, (2020, May 11). Record global carbon dioxide concentrations despite COVID-19 crisis. Retrieved from https://www.unenvironment.org/news-and-stories/story/record-global-carbon-dioxide-concentrations-despite-COVID-19-crisis

Vaughn, J. (2011). *Environmental politics: Domestic and global dimensions* (Sixth Edition) Boston: Wadsworth.

Victor, D. (2019, March 18). Dead whale found with 88 pounds of plastic inside body in the Philippines. *The New York Times*. Retrieved from https://www.nytimes.com/2019/03/18/world/asia/whale-plastics-philippines.html

WHO (n.d.) Ambient air pollution: Health impacts. Retrieved from https://www.who.int/airpollution/ambient/health-impacts/en/

Website

https://www.google.com/covid19/mobility/

6

COVID-19 and Regional Cooperation in South Asia: Challenges and Possibilities

ABSTRACT

As a global pandemic, COVID-19 crisis makes a strong case for transnational cooperation. Multilateral initiatives are imperatives that could contribute to deal with its challenge. Given the existing global trends towards parochialism and xenophobia, many argue that COVID-19 will bring strong nationalism, restrict cooperation, and embrace protectionist policies and measures. Against this backdrop, this chapter argues that it is an inescapable imperative that South Asia focus on regional cooperation to effectively deal with the multidimensional challenges of COVID-19. This chapter focuses on the role of regional cooperation in promoting and securing South Asian human security in the context of COVID-19.

Keywords: *COVID-19, Regional Cooperation, BIMSTEC, SAARC, South Asia.*

Introduction

South Asia has been witnessing onslaughts of the COVID-19 pandemic crisis. India, Pakistan, and Bangladesh have demonstrated a rampant spread of the coronavirus pandemic where about 900,000 people have been already infected. With a population of more than 1.8 billion, the region is poised to see a rising number in the coming days. Different sectors of human security in South Asia have severely been affected due to COVID-19. People are suffering from the pandemic on an unprecedented scale as several studies have revealed. The impact of COVID-19 on the poorest of the poor, low income, informal sector workers, minority groups, women and children, and vulnerable groups is colossal. A new process of pauperisation and marginalisation has begun in both developed and developing areas in the world. South Asia is particularly vulnerable to the COVID-19 pandemic due to the prevailing conditions and magnitude of poverty, inequality, and injustice in their societies. Besides, the region has not developed strong and robust national health care systems over the decades. Ironically, it has one of the lowest allocations for the healthcare sector in the world.

Analysts often express the pessimistic view that in South Asia, the fight against the virus seems to be lost before it has even begun, largely due to its poor healthcare systems. The COVID-19 not only poses a major challenge to the failing healthcare systems in the region but also to its entirety of polity, economy, and society. The economic damage, as indicated in chapter four, is immense. The predicted decline of regional GDP growth rate from an average 6.3 per cent to between 2.8 and 1.8 percent is a reality (*Dhaka Tribune*, 12 April 2020). The situation may worsen further if COVID-19 continues to hit in more than one wave. It has already increased the levels of poverty and inequality in the region. The idea of 'New Normal' captures a broad spectrum of change that is anticipated due to COVID-19 on people in South Asia. The truth is that COVID-19 has questioned the existing systems and practices in the region in organising collective actions. South Asia has been struggling to deal with the biggest challenges after it became decolonised in the late 1940s. Three major economic powers in South Asia—India, Bangladesh and Pakistan—are facing the brunt of economic mayhem caused by COVID-19.

The region has already responded to the COVID-19 crisis by declaring stimulus packages for different groups of affected people and business firms. The region has also responded in terms of healthcare services, preventive measures, redesigning administrative and bureaucratic services. While national initiatives are necessary to address the unprecedented difficulties, there is a need for embarking on initiatives to harness multilateral cooperation. Historically, global cooperation has benefitted the world to overcome challenges in peace and war alike in different phases. Challenges from any corner or any source—political, security, economic, environmental, and social—drew an immense global response in the form of dialogue, negotiations, diplomacy, and institutionalisation. Issues such as poverty, nuclear proliferation, war, climate change, trade disputes, political crisis, terrorism, war crimes, apartheid, diseases like HIV Aids, SARS and Ebola, and external aggression and so on have established widely recognised multilateral initiatives. The United Nations system is the biggest achievement of multilateral cooperation in human history. Regional cooperation is one of the effective forms of multilateral initiatives promoted by the states. The European Union (EU) and the Association of Southeast Asian Nations (ASEAN) are widely cited as the most successful examples of regional cooperation that have resolved innumerable issues and concerns in their respective regions.

Against this backdrop, this chapter attempts to understand the possibilities and challenges in dealing with the COVID-19 pandemic through South Asian regional cooperation. The nature of threats and difficulties that COVID-19 has created for the people in South Asia from a human security perspective demand collective actions at the regional level. Pandemics are, by nature, transnational threats. They have no regard for borders, and no single country can combat them alone. This chapter argues that the COVID-19 pandemic creates new ground for South Asian nations to forget their differences and strengthen regional cooperation in order to address its effects on the economy, health, and environment. It may be argued that South Asian countries have already developed a strong basis of institutional mechanisms to deal with regional challenges in development and security.

This chapter has six sections, including introduction and conclusion. In the introduction, the background and purpose of research are introduced. The second section provides an analysis of the growth of regional cooperation in South Asia. It highlights the major aspects and dynamics of the South Asian regional integration process. The third section investigates the relevance of regional response in addressing the challenge of the COVID-19 pandemic. The fourth section introduces the initiatives by the South Asian countries to organise collective action in the region in the wake of the attacks of COVID-19. The fifth section critically examines the possibilities and challenges in developing a regional response in South Asia. It demonstrates how the region can benefit from regional initiatives under SAARC or BIMSTEC. In the conclusion, it is argued that the role of India and China is extremely critical for an effective regional cooperation process in South Asia.

An Overview of Growth of Cooperation in South Asia

The narratives of regional cooperation in South Asia are old and diverse. Although the first concrete proposal for establishing a framework for regional cooperation in South Asia was made by Bangladesh in 1980, the idea of regional integration has roots in the larger dimension of Asian regionalism, which came from Japan in the late 1930s and was supported by fellow Asian people. The Japanese slogan of "Asia for the Asians" influenced the minds of colonised peoples in Asia despite the Japanese motivations being imperialistic as demonstrated during the World War II (Muni and Muni 1983: 10). Former Indian Prime Minister Nehru cherished a vision for a common platform across national boundaries. Just two years before India's freedom, Nehru said in August 1945: "I stand for a South Asian Federation of India, Iran, Iraq, Afghanistan, and Burma" (Muni and Muni 1983: 10). The issue of regional cooperation involving some South Asian countries was discussed in several conferences during 1947-1955. Some of the major conferences are the Asian Relations Conference in New Delhi in March 1947, the Baguio Conference in the Philippines in May 1950, the Colombo Plan in July 1951, and the Colombo Powers Conference in April 1954. India, Pakistan, and Sri Lanka from South Asia were co-sponsors of the historic Bandung Conference in 1955 along with Indonesia and Myanmar (Burma). Therefore, the early attempts at regionalism involving South Asian countries were connected with the larger process of Asian regionalism.

Some argue that the idea of regionalism can be traced back to early a 1976 informal gathering of scholars working on development problems. However, since 1977, Bangladesh seemed to have been working on the idea of an ASEAN-like organisation in South Asia (Hossain 2010: 134). While the Bangladesh proposal was promptly endorsed by Nepal, the Maldives, Sri Lanka and Bhutan, two countries, namely, India and Pakistan were sceptical at the outset. India's main concern was the proposal's reference to security matters in South Asia (Dash 1996). Indian policy makers also feared that Bangladesh's proposal for a regional organisation might provide an opportunity for the small neighbours to regionalise all bilateral issues and join each other to "gang up" against India. Pakistan assumed that it might be an Indian strategy to organise the other South Asian countries against Pakistan and ensure a regional market for Indian products, thereby consolidating and further strengthening India's economic dominance in the region (Dash 1996). However, subsequently, India and Pakistan changed their views and supported the regional institution-building process. During the Dhaka meeting of foreign ministers', the name of the organisation was changed from South Asian Regional Cooperation (SARC) to South Asian Association for Regional Cooperation (SAARC).

It is only in 1985 the South Asian countries formed a regional organisation called SAARC comprising seven countries such as Bangladesh, Bhutan, India, Maldives, Nepal, Pakistan, and Sri Lanka. The first summit meeting of the heads of state or government of the South Asian countries was held in Dhaka from December 7-8, 1985. Despite SAARC's slow progress and modest achievements over the past decades, the ratification of SAARC Preferential Trading Arrangement (SAPTA) by all SAARC members in December 1995 and the signing of a South Asian Free Trade Agreement (SAFTA) in January 2004 have generated guarded optimism about the relevance of SAARC in promoting regionalism in South Asia. In fact, through its Islamabad Summit in 2004, the organisation took a resolution to break down regional trade frontiers from 2006 to create a free trade zone in one of the world's most populous and poorest regions.

To identify the factors, which prompted South Asia to go for establishing a regional organisation called SAARC, it is generally viewed that the emergence of regionalism in this region did not follow the traditional arguments. During the Cold War era, many analysts argued that regionalism developed because of four conditions such as (i) common threat perception, (ii) common foreign policy orientations, (iii) presence of pivotal power, and (iv) commonalities in historical backgrounds (Ayoob 1985; Hossain 2010: 135). Some more common criteria include geographical proximity, sense of identity, interactions, and commonness. Some also argue that there are necessary and sufficient conditions for defining a regional subsystem: general geographic proximity, regularity, and intensity of interactions and shared perceptions of the regional subsystem as a distinct theatre of operations (Katzenstein 1996). In spite of fulfilling many of these attributes, South Asia remained without a regional organisation until 1985. The evolution of regional cooperation in South Asia has evolved through SAARC and subsequent initiatives of multilateral cooperation.

SAARC-Centrism

SAARC was established based on a functional theory of transnational cooperation. It is only with the formation of SAARC in 1985 that regionalism has taken some concrete shape in South Asia. Several studies demonstrate that regionalism or regional cooperation in South Asia is almost confined to SAARC that has formed a stereotype approach towards regional cooperation. Almost no attempts were made to identify new ways of looking at things. All kinds of studies on regionalism are centred on SAARC. The performance of SAARC as a regional organisation has mixed reactions. Popularly, observers of SAARC represent two clustered views, the optimists and pessimists, about the *raison d'etre* of SAARC in this region (Iftekharuzzaman 1989, 2002; Ahmed 2002; Bajpai 1999; Bhargava et al. 1995; Hossain 2010; Dash 1996). SAARC has created the basis of regional cooperation in South Asia. It has contributed to building regional solidarity and identity of people in the region. SAARC has created institutions for regional economic cooperation through the South Asian Free Trade Agreement (SAFTA). On the other hand, since its inception,

SAARC has been facing the sceptics who perceive SAARC as unnecessary or even as positively harmful. Some emphasise that South Asia has been the least integrated region in the world due to its failure to implement decisions. For them, SAARC will do little to facilitate economic growth in the region.

SAARC is extensively criticised for its narrow focus in the action agenda clearly demonstrated in its areas of cooperation. The overwhelming limitation identified by the group of sceptics was that SAARC members have been failing to put security, political and even substantive economic issues on the agenda. There is a lack of pragmatic measures for trade liberalisation under the framework of SAARC although SAFTA was floated in 2006. The SAARC process of trade liberalisation has been characterised by a lack of clarity of obligations, voluntary commitment to goals, no assurance of reciprocity among member economies and non-discrimination. Despite having criticism, SAARC is the only regional organisation where all the eight countries of South Asia are members.

Sub-regional/Inter-regional Cooperation

The proliferation of sub-regional/inter-regional groupings involving some of the members of SAARC has become a notable feature of regionalism in South Asia. Sub-regional cooperation is perceived as a mechanism for dynamic economic growth within and beyond nation-states entities. Based on the Growth Triangle (GT) model it is viewed as a solution to the operational problems of regional integration in South Asia (Kalam 2002: 197). In fact, some of the South Asian, countries sought to replicate the ASEAN and East Asian experiences of sub-regional cooperation. The organisational form of sub-regional cooperation began with the establishment of the South Asian Growth Quadrangle (SAGQ). Some states of South Asia also signed inter-regional cooperation initiatives such as the Bay of Bengal Initiative for Multi-Sectoral Technical and Economic Cooperation (BIMST-EC), South Asian Sub-regional Economic Cooperation (SASEC), Bangladesh, Bhutan, India and Nepal (BBIN), Bangladesh, Bhutan and Nepal (BBN), Bangladesh, India and Nepal (BIN),

Indian Ocean Rim Association (IORA), ASEAN Regional Forum (ARF), and Economic Cooperation Organisation (ECO). However, so far, these sub-regional and inter-regional organisations and initiatives have raised more questions, concerns, and political debate than providing answers or creating growth mechanisms and cooperative understanding.

Low Level of Economic Integration

Despite the operations of regional, sub-regional, and inter-regional cooperative frameworks in South Asia, economic integration remains at a low level. Even the establishment of the South Asian Preferential Trading Arrangement (SAPTA) in 1995 in order to augment intra-SAARC trade in this region has failed to create a momentum for economic integration. Later, the South Asian Trade Agreement (SAFTA) was signed and came into force in January 2006 after several rounds of trade negotiations. SAFTA has remained equally ineffective in South Asia. Such a low level of economic integration may be attributed to the failure of SAARC member countries in incorporating substantive economic issues at the formative state of regional cooperation. The historical missing of economic agenda in SAARC deliberations since its inception hindered the growth of meaningful cooperation in the economic arena.

Politico-Strategic Cooperation

Although it is not under the purview of the SAARC framework to contribute to political and strategic cooperation in South Asia, it was expected that the so-called spillover effect could have some positive impact on the on-going scenarios. It is well known that SAARC has practically done nothing in this field. No regional initiative within or beyond SAARC as seen in the case of the trade arena was taken or even envisaged by the South Asian leaders. As Sabur (2002:74) points out, the concrete achievements of SAARC, in terms of fostering either regional cooperation or friendly relations among the member states were insignificant. The politico-security environment in South Asia remains full of suspicion, mistrust, and hostility. Bilateral disputes have constantly overshadowed the process of regional cooperation within the framework of SAARC. As a result, the overall security environment remains unchanged; perhaps it has gone from bad to worse. The nuclear tests in May 1999 by India and Pakistan trigger a further blow to the already existing worsening situation. The nuclearisation of South Asia associated with the arms race, Kashmir conflict, post-9/11 syndromes, and a host of bilateral disputes show deteriorating regional strategic scenarios.

It may be mentioned here that both India and Pakistan have diametrically opposite strategic postures based on divergent threat perceptions. The Indian strategic posture is deeply influenced by the so-called 'India Doctrine' wherein India perceives South Asia as its periphery in relations to its strategic linkages with the neighbouring countries. Under such a scheme, India views the entire region as a single strategic unit and herself as its sole custodian of security and stability (Iftekharuzzaman 1989). Pakistan, as the chief contender of India's security doctrine, remains committed to facing India under any circumstances. The arms build-up in Pakistan and the pursuit of extra-regional military cooperation play a vital role in this regard. Though the smaller members of South Asia are the champions of regional cooperation, for that matter, regionalism, they are also in conflict with India and Pakistan.

Role of Civil Society
Long neglected as a force of change, civil society has vigorously come to the forefront of national, regional, and global domains of human activities. South Asian leaders now recognise that social forces outside the purview of governments can play a constructive role in consolidating regional cooperation. The justification pertains to two major factors. On the one hand, the governments in South Asia have consistently been failing to deliver goods to the people. The frequent postponements of Summits, the display of deep mistrust and suspicion while they negotiate, inability to crack new grounds of cooperation in substantive areas and, above all, the lack of dynamism put the governments on trial about the future of regionalism in South Asia. On the other hand, the agenda of regional cooperation through SAARC reflects a wide range of social, cultural, and economic aspects affecting the life and welfare of the citizens (Iftekharuzzaman 2002: 25). NGOs are considered as infrastructure for

regional cooperation, particularly in the process of confidence-building measures (CBMs) and security dialogues. The fact remains that when the role of civil society is strongly envisaged, it is not to discard or substitute governments; instead, it is to assert their own role in the process and thereby influence organisational performance.

Regionalism and Globalisation

Regionalism in South in its current form has not been able to embrace the most recent global phenomenon known as 'globalisation' whereas it has generated enormous pressures on nation-states individually and regionally. The political, economic, cultural, and security foundations of globalisation have created a new condition for the survival of humankind. Accountability, decentralisation, civil society, and popular participation have become important to explain social phenomena in the age of globalisation. Economic globalisation appears more significant in terms of its impact on the power and legitimacy of the state and state system, which grants a new kind of structural power to capital over labour in countries around the world. Various forces behind the process of globalisation such as financial openness, privatisation, trade liberalisation, democratisation, civil society empowerment and information and communication technology (ICT) have been contributing to far-reaching global changes.

Against such a backdrop, different regions responded to the globalisation process in different ways depending on their economic capacity, trade opportunities, access to finance, and orientations of the states that form the region. In the face of structural changes at the global level, regionalisation, therefore, emerged to maximise trade benefits, or as new forms of collaboration to stimulate growth (Rahman 1999). The examples of the European Union (EU), Association of Southeast Asian Nations (ASEAN), North American Free Trade Agreement (NAFTA), Asia Pacific Economic Cooperation (APEC) and many more can be mentioned. The growth of regional cooperation in South Asia shows that member-countries are strongly engaged in different institutional architectures for multilateral cooperation. SAARC, BIMSTEC, BCIM, SASEC, and BBIN are the major organisational forms, which have the potential for building cooperation on the issue of the COVID-19 pandemic.

Relevance of Regional Response to COVID-19

> Voila, suddenly, entirely unexpectedly, we now have that external enemy, the COVID-19, which has already most tellingly demonstrated, in its most insidious way, its perilous propensity for replicating, mutating, propagating and attacking, making no distinction whatever among race, class, caste, religion, gender, nationality and geo-spatial location. We are all today confronted with a very dangerous pandemic that could pose an existential threat to governments, regimes and peoples across the region in yet unimagined ways (Karim 2020).

Despite the poor performance of South Asian countries in utilising regional integration for resolving collective action problems, it is always relevant to the policy choices of member-nations. South Asia is institutionally equipped to deal with transnational threats like the COVID-19 pandemic. On the one hand, members of the South Asian region have their own regional and sub-regional initiatives such as SAARC, SAFTA, SASEC, and BBIN. On the other hand, South Asian countries are associated with several inter-regional and sub-regional cooperation organisations such as BIMSTEC, BCIM, IORA, ASEAN Regional Forum (ARF), and ECO. South Asian countries are poised to mobilise regional resources and initiatives to support actions for fighting the COVID-19 pandemic. It is the political will of the member-nations that can engage these countries in promoting a regional response to COVID-19. The relevance of such a response in the case of South Asia may be considered for a number of reasons.

First and foremost, the COVID-19 pandemic is, by nature, a transnational threat that needs regional and global initiatives for effective response strategies. South Asian countries can join together to identify proper measures in this extraordinary time. In the words of Tariq Karim, 'There is nothing like a good common existential threat to all of us to make us focus on that threat, to collectively and in concert endeavour to combat, contain and overcome it decisively' (Karim 2020). Second, the nature of the effects of COVID-19 for South Asia is common to the whole region. The entire region is characterised by common challenges such as poverty, inequality, and injustice. The COVID-19 pandemic has exacerbated these issues in the region. The number of poor people has already doubled in the region. Even the macroeconomic challenges are also common such as loss of revenue, shrinking of exports and a sharp decline in GDP growth rate. Third, South Asia has already developed regional mechanisms that can be applied in the case of the COVID-19 pandemic. As mentioned above, SAARC and BIMSTEC could be effective platforms for a regional response to the crisis.

Fourth, South Asia may benefit from the regional response with a specific focus on health issues. The national health systems are not in good shape in most of the South Asian countries. In such a crisis, both the public and private health systems fail. During this crisis, South Asian countries can explore the use of the pool of doctors, nurses, and medical facilities available in this region to help each other. Previously, SAARC created a forum of meeting for SAARC health ministers in the wake of the outbreak of the Severe Acute Respiratory Syndrome (SARS). It was an emergency meeting of SAARC Health Ministers, which was held in Male in April 2003 to develop a regional strategy to deal with the deadly epidemic. Meanwhile, there were six meetings of the SAARC health ministers held between 2003 and 2017.

Fifth, South Asian countries need to share their experiences of the national policy measures to combat the COVID-19 crisis. Different countries in the region have already responded to the crisis by declaring stimulus packages targeting the vulnerable people and business sectors. Sixth, against the backdrop of disruptions in the global supply chains for a large number of sectors, South Asian countries need to explore the use of regional supply chains as much as possible. The COVID-19 crisis demonstrates that the overwhelming dependence on a few countries, both in the cases of exports and imports, is counterproductive (Raihan 2020).

Seventh, SAARC and BIMSTEC leaders have a new opportunity to rejuvenate the regional cooperation process. SAARC remains dormant since the postponement of the 19th Islamabad Summit due to be held in

November 2016. Although BIMSTEC has been relatively visible over the last five years, it requires new impetus to energise its functioning process. The crisis brought about by COVID-19 can lead to an understanding of the need for greater transnational cooperation through SAARC and BIMSTEC processes and crafting new measures to put aside their differences in South Asia. The collective endeavours for vaccines, finding ways for dealing with common economic challenges and building a peaceful atmosphere clearly focus on a regional response. Last, but not the least, David Brewster rightly argues that the COVID-19 pandemic crisis has implications for regional security and regional relationships which may endure in different degrees for several years in different regions including South Asia (Brewster 2020).

COVID-19 Focused Initiatives

As a surprise to observers of South Asian regional cooperation, leaders in South Asia have already come forward to address the COVID-19 crisis through a regional platform. The Prime Minister of India, Narendra Modi, proposed a virtual summit of SAARC leaders in the beginning of the COVID-19 pandemic in South Asia. All the member-nations responded to the initiative positively. The virtual video-summit was held on 16 March 2020. During the summit, the Indian prime minister proposed an emergency COVID-19 fund for SAARC countries, emphasised reviving of the SAARC FINANCE Forum to discuss how this emergency fund could be created, expanded, and used.

Rajiv Bhatia summarises the achievements of the first ever-virtual summit quite well. In his view, the initiative of the SAARC virtual summit is significant for a number of reasons (Bhatia 2020). First, for the first time since 2016, all the eight-member nations joined at a conference of heads of states or governments, except Pakistan. The Secretary-General of SAARC also joined the conference, which has agreed to work jointly to contain COVID-19 and shared their perspectives and experiences. Second, India has proposed to launch a COVID-19 Emergency Fund that received a positive nod from members. All member-nations except Pakistan have already contributed voluntarily to the total amount of US$ 18.8 million.

Third, it was decided that each contributing member would approve and disburse in response to requests from others. Fourth, India has played a leading role in mobilising the fund with its initial contribution of US$ 10 million. Finally, follow-up initiatives are also visible in connection with the Summit.

In the follow-up period, the first video-conference of senior health officials was arranged on March 26, 2020. The agenda included issues ranging from specific protocols dealing with screening at entry points and contact tracing to online training capsules for emergency response teams (Bhatia 2020). Eventually, the second video conference of health ministers of SAARC member-states was held on March 27, 2020. A third e-conference of SAARC trade officials was convened on April 8, 2020 to assess the implications of COVID-19 for intra-regional trade stemming from travel restrictions.

Apart from the creation of the Emergency Fund, SAARC leaders agreed to undertake several measures such as the creation of Rapid Response Teams for COVID-19, Online Training Capsules, holding Video Conference of Doctors, Video Conference of Trade Officials, launching COVID Website, Integrated Health Platform for Disease Surveillance and creation of Research Platforms. Each member-state designated its national focal points of SAARC at Foreign Ministries as the SAARC COVID-19 Focal Point (MOFA, Bangladesh n.d.). Bangladesh proposed to host a research institute to fight future public health threats in the SAARC region. As part of the regional initiative, India has sent emergency medical assistance consisting of 30,000 RT-PCR COVID-19 test kits to Bangladesh (*The Daily Star*, 6 May 2020). India has already started using the fund to send medical assistance to Afghanistan, Bhutan, and Nepal.

Besides, the World Economic Forum (WEF) has mobilised South Asian policymakers through a COVID-19 regional action group. Functional challenges such as migration and food production are being addressed as part of Track II cooperation. (Ibrahimi and Kamal 2020). Universities, think-tanks and civil society organisations also arranged several virtual meetings and conferences focusing on regional scenarios in South Asia centring on the COVID-19 challenge. South Asian scholars and activists have joined these regional initiatives.

The perspectives and initiatives of BIMSTEC are also important to understand the South Asian response to the COVID-19 challenge. Given the scope and areas of cooperation of BIMSTEC, the organisation is in a great position to support the member-countries fighting against the COVID-19 challenge. BIMSTEC is a sector-driven cooperation forum where specific issues such as public health, trade and connectivity may be addressed with strong collective measures. It is heartening to observe that the Secretary-General of BIMSTEC, Shahidul Islam, strongly established a case for considering COVID-19 challenges by the members of the organisations. Since there are five South Asian nations as members of BIMSTEC, it can contribute to enhancing a regional response. In the words of Islam, 'As the pandemic increasingly transforms itself into an economic crisis, the areas of cooperation identified by BIMSTEC appears to be equally relevant in the post-COVID-19 era; the only difference is that we will need to do the same work in a better way and at a faster pace' (Islam 2020).

On the occasion of the 23rd BIMSTEC Day, heads of the governments and states of BIMSTEC have shared highly optimistic ideas to cooperate in the time of the COVID-19 crisis and its aftermath. The Prime Minister of Bangladesh, Sheikh Hasina, spells out, 'Bimstec forum provides an excellent platform to combat the devastating impact of COVID-19. We should not leave any stone unturned to utilise this platform in addressing the challenges of the post-COVID-19 era' (*Dhaka Tribune*, June 5, 2020). Similarly, the Prime Minister of India, Narendra Modi, expressed the need for regional cooperation: 'The world is currently fighting the common challenge of COVID-19 pandemic. No individual country can, by itself, overcome its huge consequences. In our common endeavour to deal with this unprecedented threat, India stands ready to share its expertise, resources, capacities and knowledge with all countries in the region' (*Dhaka Tribune*, June 5, 2020). These words from BIMSTEC leaders are a reflection of the clear policy direction towards a regional response to the COVID-19 crisis.

New Prospects and Old Challenges

The virtual summit of SAARC and the statements of BIMSTEC leaders have clearly transmitted a positive message to the people in South Asia that a regional response to fight against the COVID-19 challenge is urgently needed. It has created a new occasion to be seized upon by the South Asian leaders amid the COVID-19 pandemic crisis. National, bilateral and global measures as relevant to South Asia are not adequate. COVID-19-based regional cooperation has a huge prospect to complement the national efforts of South Asian countries. What are the reasons behind a new prospect of regional cooperation centring on COVID-19 pandemic? Seven points are pertinent to understand this question.

First, the national response to the COVID-19 crisis through stimulus packages and a plethora of preventive and protective measures are not simply enough as indicated in section three. Analysts argue that challenges remain due to limited resources at the disposal of governments. It has already been announced that India has pumped a $ 23 billion stimulus package into its economy to sustain over 1 billion people. In comparison, Germany is pouring in 750 billion Euros ($ 815 billion) into its economy with a population of 83 million. Bangladesh's stimulus package is US$ 11.5 billion equivalent 3.3 per cent of GDP (Ibrahimi and Kamal 2020). Governments in South Asia have already asked for external support from donors to support them to meet the COVID-19 challenge. For example, the World Bank has already allocated $ 1.4 billion in aid for South Asian countries to tackle this problem. Pakistan has asked for debt relief for all developing countries in the wake of this catastrophe, which will be essential for the revival of the economies in the region (Ibrahimi and Kamal 2020). Besides, South Asian countries have been struggling with their limited resources and capacity to supply necessary medical treatment, equipment and logistics for 1.8 billion people.

Second, the initiatives that have been undertaken so far demonstrate an urgency from South Asian leaders to rely on the regional cooperation process in order to face the new challenge created by COVID-19. For a region known to the world as one of the least integrated of its kind, these initiatives certainly generate a hope. The concrete measures as mulled through the virtual summit of SAARC countries are significant in the current context. The emergency COVID-19 fund, e-conferences of health ministers, e-meetings of trade officials and a regional website for COVID-19 are beneficial for the people in the region. The SAARC Comprehensive Framework on Disaster Management provides a roadmap for cooperation in natural disasters including pandemics like COVID-19 (Wignaraja et al. 2020). Panditaratne argues, 'SAARC could prioritise medical treatment of COVID to ensure that any eventual vaccine or any eventual medical treatment is accessible throughout South Asia as opposed to in the production centres' (Varma 2020). BIMSTEC's perspective on the COVID-19 pandemic is also critically important to identify new measures under this organisation.

Third, national health systems in South Asia are underdeveloped and vulnerable which has become abundantly clear during the COVID-19 crisis. Particularly, public health systems in the region are in deep crisis. Citizens in the region have expressed utter dismay about corruption, irregularities, mismanagement and lack of resources in different countries. Given such weak systems of public health, regional cooperation becomes an imperative for the member-nations.

Fourth, poverty and inequality in the region have always been major causes behind regional cooperation in South Asia and these have been overlooked by the leaders. Now due to the COVID-19 pandemic, people in South Asia are witnessing rising trends towards further pauperisation and marginalisation. Millions of low wage and informal sector workers, low and middle-income people, and vulnerable groups have been suffering from acute shortages of support from the governments and society. This necessitates regional endeavours focusing on the initiatives, which have already been spelled out by the region.

Fifth, South Asia may benefit from the attention of the major powers, particularly in the current context of social and health crisis created by COVID-19. The region is becoming increasingly contested for influence by China, which has implications for the regional strategic environment.

It may be argued that extra regional powers such as the United States of America (USA), China, Japan and the EU may present opportunities to extend the benefits of economic development and invest in supply chains and increased connectivity for goods and services (Samaranayake 2020). The leadership from South Asia could exploit this new global attention to the region for the welfare of more than 20 per cent global population living in South Asia.

Sixth, India's outreach to South Asian countries may be considered a gesture and prospect that could eventually lead to some positive outcomes. India's approach has been proactive since the outbreak of the crisis. India's initiative to convene a virtual summit of SAARC and supporting South Asian countries in evacuating citizens from Wuhan, China, the epicentre of the first COVID-19 outbreak, are cases in point. India has emerged as a major supplier of medicines to different countries worldwide in the fight against COVID-19, which may be strength for South Asia as a source of life-saving medicines (Marjani 2020). Finally, South Asia cannot remain isolated from the practices as observed in different regions in the world. For example, the EU has created the Coronavirus Response Investment Initiative, which has received 37 billion Euros to support the hardest hit member-states to get access to financial support. The EU has also launched a 750 billion Euro Pandemic Emergency Purchase Programme (PEPP) as a bailout measure for the member-nations that would enable them to absorb the carbon shock (Ghosh 2020).

While the prospects for regional cooperation in the COVID-19 era are evident, the challenges are manifold. These are the age-old challenges in South Asia, which are intrinsically linked with geopolitical considerations. Any effective regional cooperation initiative faces at least five challenges in South Asia.

First and foremost, India-Pakistan rivalry has been a major stumbling block to the regional cooperation process through SAARC or BIMSTEC. Since its creation in 1985, SAARC faced the dilemma of dealing with two rival powers—India and Pakistan. Summits have been postponed one after another largely due to India-Pakistan hostility. In its thirty-five years of history, SAARC could hold only eighteen summits. The current impasse in SAARC on the question of holding the 19th Summit emanates primarily from this reality.

Second, another major geopolitical challenge that is relatively recent is China-India rivalry. The fallouts of China's Belt and Road Initiative (BRI), Indo Pacific Strategy (IPS), Sino-Indian Doklam standoff in 2017 and border skirmishes in May 2020 have changed the strategic priorities of India as the dominant actor in South Asia. Both BIMSTEC and SAARC suffer from these two strategic challenges as they are deeply connected with traditional security concerns.

Third, bilateral relations between Pakistan and Bangladesh and Pakistan and Afghanistan have created a new front of strategic difficulty in South Asia. Pakistan's attempt to interfere in the domestic affairs of Bangladesh and historical differences between the two countries based on the Liberation War of Bangladesh in 1971 have worsened their bilateral relations in recent years. Insurgency, terrorism, border dispute, the Taliban issue and the India factor have bedevilled Pakistan-Afghanistan relations in the post-9/11 era.

Fourth, there is a tendency for making BIMSTEC an alternative to the SAARC pushed by India. This is a perception generally shared by member-countries of South Asia (Varma 2020). Finally, the ensuing cold war between the USA and China has its strategic impact on South Asia as the entire region is closely linked with these two global powers. The policy priorities of smaller countries in South Asian are often at odds with Sino-Indian and Sino-US rivalries, which has complicated the politico-strategic dimensions of South Asia. Pakistan's alliance type relations with China as demonstrated through the controversial China-Pakistan Economic Corridor (CPEC) have added further difficulty in strategic environment.

The regional dynamics in South Asia and neighbouring regions demonstrate both possibilities and challenges in consolidating the regional cooperation process to deal with the COVID-19 crisis. While challenges are there, the prospects for regional cooperation are immense. It is true that SAARC is caught into a technical mess due to its inability to hold the 19th Summit scheduled in 2016, but it has different institutional mechanisms in place for generating a regional response. This has already become evident as indicated above. It is an occasion for the region to move beyond nationalist sentiments and geopolitical fault lines. Moreover, many in South Asia question the existing paradigm where the peoples are facing a reality of high transaction costs and a regression to a devastated Hobbesian state that Europe witnessed at the end of World War II. South Asia can no longer endure the burden of the inconceivable costs of non-cooperation.

Conclusion

This chapter has investigated the possibilities and hurdles for regional cooperation that South Asia desperately needs to consider in the time of the global pandemic called COVID-19. It has demonstrated the relevance of a regional response to face the COVID-19 challenge in an effective way. It is emphasised that regional cooperation can provide additional avenue to respond to the pandemic, by establishing regional and/or sub-regional initiatives as seen in the case of the EU. Specifically, South Asia may benefit from regional cooperation through a public health emergency fund and coordinating debt relief measures. South Asia has already developed strong institutional mechanisms to create a regional response to face any social and economic crisis in the region. SAARC, as the oldest regional endeavour along with BIMSTEC, could have a significant impact on deciding the positive directions toward a common stance on COVID-19. This study has argued that there is a genuine rationale behind the relevance of regional response in South Asia. It has also specified the areas where South Asian leaders could find a real prospect for engagement in supporting the regional cooperation process. This chapter has also emphasised that it is not only SAARC that can lead the process, but BIMSTEC can also play a critical role.

Considering the urgency of regional cooperation and ensuing geopolitical challenges, it is emphatically argued that India and China have a critical role in the entire process. The COVID-19 pandemic has created a humanitarian situation for the entire world including South Asia. With a poor record of human security in South Asia, regional leaders are compelled to rise to the occasion forgetting their differences and narrow geopolitical calculations. Both China and India could choose to use the COVID-19 crisis to find areas for enhanced cooperation in a new and reshaped post-COVID-19 world order (Brewster 2020). It is widely recognised that China is a "physical infrastructure provider" while India is a "digital infrastructure provider" in the form of e-commerce, Internet penetration, mobile, and smart-phone rates (Varma 2020). This is a synergy that South Asia is in great need to address the COVID-19 crisis.

India's role is specifically vital to the whole process. Analysts point out that India as the dominant country in the region and as part of her Neighbourhood First policy must come forward to rediscover regional solidarity and cohesion in South Asia. India has demonstrated its willingness in such an endeavour by calling the first ever virtual summit of SAARC on 12 March 2020 in order to formulate a regional strategy against the challenge of COVID-19. Besides, India could take an initiative and become a major supplier of testing kits, as the region stands suspicious of Chinese kits (Varma 2020).

India has also a geopolitical reason behind its regional leadership in post-pandemic rehabilitation. It is widely known that China has been expanding its influence in South Asia and could step in more aggressively to assist weakened states to control them in the future. India could emerge ahead in the contest with China with the right mix of policies (Haqqani and Pande 2020). Overall, India deserves a central role given its size and "role as a magnet that attracts attention from around the world" (Varma 2020). In the absence of a solid and mutually beneficial regional cooperation process, the rest of South Asia would move away from the path of regional integration and toward China. China is the largest trade partner of Bangladesh and Pakistan while Sri Lanka's trade relationship with China has grown rapidly in recent times. In fact, China surpassed India as Sri Lanka's biggest import partner in 2018, another sign of China's growing influence in South Asia.

Although China is an extra-regional power, the country has deeply been engaged in South Asia. Particularly its economic engagement is high in all countries including India. The volume of Sino-Indian trade is US$ 84.38 billion (Bhowmick 2020). Interestingly, unlike other major powers in Asia, China is not heavily connected with regional and sub-regional processes. China is an observer of SAARC that gives an institutional basis to engage in the South Asian regional cooperation process. China has the advantage of its larger foreign currency reserves and the ability to offer loans and investment (Haqqani and Pande 2020). China has developed a powerful platform such as BRI to engage South Asian countries through connectivity and trade. However, the pursuit of China in bilateral engagement creates more geopolitical risks and eventually complicates the environment detrimental to its interests. China must play a positive role in promoting regional cooperation in South Asia. Its Pakistan-focused policy should be reconsidered to restore trust and confidence in the region, which will ensure mutual benefits for all.

In conclusion, this chapter argues that it is time for countries in South Asia to demonstrate a true spirit of resilience and find ways to use the COVID-19 pandemic as an opportunity for consolidating regional integration. In this context, the leaders in the region must shun the politics of divisions and xenophobia, shelve interstate disputes, and allow international organisations, civil society, the private sector, and philanthropists to play their roles.

REFERENCES

Ahmed, I. (2002, January 1). Between regionalism and the nation-state: The Himal Roundtable on Re-Conceptualizing South Asia. *Himal Southasia*. Retrieved from https://www.himalmag.com/between-regionalism-and-the-nation-state/

Ayoob, M. (1985). The primacy of the political: South Asian regional cooperation in comparative perspective. A paper presented at the International Conference on *South Asian Regional Cooperation*, Organized by BIISS, Dhaka, 14-16 January.

Bajpai, K. (1999). Security and SAARC. In E. Gonsalves and N. Jetly (eds.), *The dynamics of South Asia: Regional cooperation and SAARC*, New Delhi: Vedams Books.

Bhargava, K. K.; Bongartz, H. & Sobhan, F. (eds.), (1995). *Shaping South Asia's future: Role of regional cooperation*. New Delhi: Vikas Publishing House Pvt. Ltd.

Bhatia, R. (2020, April 7). Preparing for SAARC 2.0, *The Hindu*. Retrieved from https://www.thehindu.com/opinion/op-ed/preparing-for-saarc-20/article31273813.ece

Bhowmick, S. (2020, March 26). Reimagining BIMSTEC amidst the COVID-19 disaster. Observer Research Foundation, India. Retrieved from https://www.orfonline.org/expert-speak/reimagining-bimstec-amidst-the-COVID-19-disaster-63736/

Brewster, D. (2020, April 10). Why South Asia may come out of COVID-19 crisis better than many expect. *The Interpreter*. Retrieved from https://www.lowyinstitute.org/the-interpreter/why-south-asia-may-come-out-COVID-19-crisis-better-many-expect

Dash, K.C. (1996). The political economy of regional cooperation in South Asia. *Pacific Affairs*, 69(2), 185-209.

Dhaka Tribune (2020, April 12). World Bank: GDP growth to crash to 2 to 3% in FY20. Retrieved from https://www.dhakatribune.com/business/2020/04/12/wb-bangladesh-must-ramp-up-coronavirus-action-to-protect-its-people-revive-economy

Dhaka Tribune (2020, June 5). 23rd Bimstec Day: Bimstec leaders for joint efforts to combat COVID-19 impact. Retrieved from https://www.dhakatribune.com/bangladesh/foreign-affairs/2020/06/05/23rd-bimstec-day-bimstec-leaders-for-joint-efforts-to-combat-COVID-19-impact

Ghosh, P. S. (2020, May 20). Playing the COVID-19 card to sustain the SAARC nonsense. *Dhaka Tribune*. Retrieved from https://www.dhakatribune.com/opinion/op-ed/2020/05/20/playing-the-COVID-19-card-to-sustain-the-saarc-nonsense

Haqqani, H. & Pande, A. (2020, May 26). Crisis from Kolkata to Kabul: COVID-19's impact on South Asia. Hudson Institute. Retrieved from https://www.hudson.org/research/16070-crisis-from-kolkata-to-kabul-COVID-19-s-impact-on-south-asia

Hossain, D. (2010). *Globalization and new regionalism in South Asia: Issues and dynamics*. Dhaka: AH Development Publishing House.

Ibrahimi, S.S. & Kamal, S.M. (2020, April 30). The battles that can cost South Asia the war against COVID-19. *The Diplomat*. Retrieved from https://thediplomat.com/2020/04/the-battles-that-can-cost-south-asia-the-war-against-COVID-19/

Iftekharuzzaman (1989). The India doctrine: Relevance for Bangladesh. In M. G. Kabir & S. Hossain (eds.), *Issues and challenges facing Bangladesh foreign policy*, (pp.18-43), Dhaka: Bangladesh Society for International Studies.

Iftekharuzzaman (2002). Reforming SAARC: In spite of governments. In S. Afroze (ed.), *Regional cooperation in South Asia: New dimensions and perspectives* (pp.17-29), Dhaka: Bangladesh Institute of International and Strategic Studies.

Islam, S. (2020, June 6). BIMSTEC to stay course in post-COVID-19 era. *bdnews24.com*. Retrieved from https://opinion.bdnews24.com/2020/06/06/bimstec-to-stay-course-in-post-COVID-19-era/

Kalam, A. (2002). Sub-regional growth mechanisms: SAGQ and IMS-GT in comparative perspective. In S. Afroze (ed.), *Regional cooperation in South Asia: New dimensions and perspectives* (pp.173-234), Dhaka: Bangladesh Institute of International and Strategic Studies.

Karim, T. (2020, March 22). The implications of coronavirus for regional and global cooperation. *The Daily Star*. Retrieved from https://www.thedailystar.net/opinion/news/implications-coronavirus-regional-and-global-cooperation-1884058

Katzenstein, P. J. (1996). Regionalism in comparative perspective. *Cooperation and Conflict*, 31 (2), 123-159.

Marjani, N. (2020, April 22). India's Indian Ocean diplomacy in the COVID-19 crisis. *The Diplomat*. Retrieved from https://thediplomat.com/2020/04/indias-indian-ocean-diplomacy-in-the-COVID-19-crisis/

MOFA, Bangladesh. (n.d.). Regional cooperation: SAARC initiatives on COVID-19. Retrieved from https://mofa.gov.bd/site/page/9ee3e51e-29dd-4619-9088-e82a63b32a05/Regional-Cooperation

Muni, S.D. & Muni, A. (1983). *Regional cooperation in South Asia*. New Delhi: National.

Rahman, A. (1999). Beyond nation state: Globalization and regionalism in South Asia. Paper presented at regional workshop on globalization and security in South Asia, jointly organized by Bangladesh Institute of International and Strategic Studies (BIISS) and Regional Centre for Strategic Studies (RCSS), held in Dhaka during May 25-27.

Raihan, S. (2020, April 9). Case for a united South Asian response to COVID-19. *The Daily Star*. Retrieved from https://www.thedailystar.net/opinion/news/case-united-south-asian-response-COVID-19-1891000.

Sabur, A.K.M.A. (2002). Regional cooperation in South Asia: Problems of conflict management. In S. Afroze (ed.), *Regional cooperation in South Asia: New dimensions and Perspectives* (pp. 71-127), Dhaka: Bangladesh Institute of International and Strategic Studies (BIISS).

Samaranayake, N. (2020, May 6). COVID-19-and-competition-for-influence-in-south-asia. *South Asia Journal*. Retrieved from http://southasiajournal.net/COVID-19-and-competition-for-influence-in-south-asia/

The Daily Star (2020, May 6). India sends 30,000 COVID-19 test kits as part of SAARC initiative. Retrieved from https://www.thedailystar.net/india-sends-30000-COVID-19-test-kits-part-saarc-initiative-1900048

Varma, N. (2020, May 13). Webinar: Will COVID-19 reverse regional connectivity? Perspectives from South Asia. Brookings India. Retrieved from https://www.brookings.edu/events/webinar-will-COVID-19-reverse-regional-connectivity-perspectives-from-south-asia/

Wignaraja, G., Raihan, S., Sharma, P., Ahmed, V. & De, P. (2020, April 26). Five proposals to tackle COVID-19 in South Asia. *The Prospector*. Retrieved from https://lki.lk/blog/five-proposals-to-tackle-COVID-19-in-south-asia/

7

COVID-19 and the Crisis of Global Health Governance: Implications for South Asia

ABSTRACT

As disease does not respect international borders, health challenge has often been identified as a common challenge that humanity faces. And given the level of multidimensional inter-dependence and inter-connectedness between states and non-state actors, one state's health challenge surpasses easily across borders, which creates vulnerability for other states. Thus, global health governance becomes essential. Against this backdrop, this chapter investigates three questions: What factors have led to the failure of global health governance in addressing the COVID-19 global pandemic? What would be the implications of global health governance in case of failure for South Asia? What can be done to strengthen global health governance in the post-COVID-19 era? This chapter argues that non-cooperation, the crisis of global leadership, the marginalisation of the World Health Organisation (WHO), the marginalisation of science from policy processes have contributed to the failure of global health governance. Indeed, the indispensable role of global health governance needs to be acknowledged and embraced by the major powers in the domain of world politics for the betterment of the people. It is only possible when people and the WHO would be the priority area of world politics. Thus, this chapter presents a case for strengthening the World Health Organisation for better global health governance.

Keywords: *COVID-19, Global Health Governance, World Health Organisation, International Cooperation.*

Introduction

> *We've learned that yours is the first generation in global history where the fate of everyone—all 7.7 billion people in 195 nation states—is truly linked as never before. That is what the coronavirus and extraordinary economic collapse have taught us this spring.*
> —**Ambassador Nicholas Burns**, May 15, 2020 (Burns 2020).

The above quotation from Ambassador Burns tells us about the interdependent world and the mutual vulnerability of health challenges that underscores the necessity of global health governance. The COVID-19 global pandemic highlights the need for global cooperation on health and thus, global health governance. As mentioned in chapter 3, COVID-19, which originated in Wuhan, spread quickly to all corners of the world with severe human (in) security implications. As of June 19, 2020, the novel coronavirus had infected 8,685,763 people and killed 459,004 people globally. No state is immune to this deadly virus. In addition, one can look at some contemporary examples to understand the need for global health governance. The 2014-15 Ebola outbreak in West Africa infected almost 30000 people and killed more than 11,000 people and led to billions of dollars of economic losses. Furthermore, one can argue that the outbreak of Middle East Respiratory Syndrome (MERS), the resurgence of polio in the Middle East, South Asia, Africa, and Ukraine and other parts of the world, the 2016 Zika virus outbreak in North America and the 2003 SARS outbreak tell us the simple story that no state can alone solve the problem of infectious diseases which bring heavy consequences for the world at large. Thus, it is argued that 'a nation's health can be effectively secured only through international cooperation' (Gostin 2017:224). But in the case of fighting COVID-19, there is a clear absence of international cooperation and coordination. In addition, it is manifested that the global health governance (GHG) institution, i.e., the World Health Organisation, has been sidelined and denied cooperation (when WHO needed cooperation badly) by the major powers, including the USA. It sends a negative signal for post-COVID-19 global health governance. But the importance of global health governance is undeniable for world peace, prosperity, security, and cooperation. In this context, this chapter merits serious attention. It mainly investigates three questions: What factors have led to the failure of global health governance in addressing the COVID-19 global pandemic? What would be the implications of global health governance failure for South Asia? What can be done to strengthen global health governance in the post-COVID-19 era?

This chapter is divided into six sections, including the introduction. In the second section, the chapter focuses on the theorisation of GHG, while the third section discusses GHG from a historical background. The fourth section examines the crisis of GHG during the COVID-19 period, and the fifth section focuses on possible policy responses. The final section concludes.

Theorising Global Health Governance

Though global health governance has become a buzzword in the twenty first century, it is very much contested. It is pertinent to look at what the terms 'global health' and 'governance' mean before theorising 'global health governance'. Simply put, 'global' refers to everything happening worldwide. And 'governance' is basically the act of governing. According to the Oxford Dictionary, governance is 'the activity of governing a country or controlling a company or an organisation; the way in which a country is governed or a company or institution is controlled'. The Commission on Global Governance in fact, defines governance as 'the sum of the many ways individuals and institutions, public and private, manage their common affairs' (Commission on Global Governance 1995:2). Dodgson et al. (2002:6) argue that 'governance can be defined as the actions and means adopted by a society to promote collective action and deliver collective solutions in pursuit of common goals...encompassing the many ways in which human beings, as individuals and groups, organise themselves to achieve agreed goals'. Health governance means the 'actions and means adopted by a society to organise itself in the promotion and protection of the health of its population' (Dodgson et al. 2002:6). It is further noted that 'the rules defining such organisation, and its functioning, can again be formal (Public Health Act, International Health

Regulations) or informal (e.g., the Hippocratic Oath) to prescribe and proscribe behaviour' (Dodgson et al. 2002:6).

Similarly, GHG has been defined as the 'shorthand for the rules, norms, and formal institutions that mediate and facilitate international interactions related to health' (Batniji and Songane 2014: 65). The functions of GHG have been identified as international financing on health, regulation, and cooperative research. Institutions play a leading role in global health governance as it is argued that 'all health problems, whether child mortality, infectious diseases, Ebola, or mental health, need institutional support and resources' (Clinton and Sridhar 2017:x).

Global health governance developed due to the growing interdependence among states and non-state actors, the development of scientific and technological knowledge over global health, and the growth of international institutions (Zacher and Keefe 2008). And scholarly interest in global health governance (GHG) began with the end of the Cold War (McInnes et al. 2014). This was partly because of the removal of the Cold War's narrow agenda (McInnes and Lee 2012) and partly because of the increased fear of infectious diseases (Garret 1996; Price-Smith 2001). Clinton and Sridhar (2017) identify three key drivers in global health governance, i.e., recognition that health challenges cross national borders, which require intergovernmental cooperation; the increasing role played by non-state actors, i.e., NGOs, foundations/philanthropies in the global governance decision-making; and increasing evidence that global challenges require efficient and equitable collective action solutions.

GHG institutions are likely to empower scientists and relatively weaker states (Batniji and Songane 2014). But in contemporary GHG, science has been marginalised and major powers'/donors' interests are prioritised at the expense of the interests of the developing world. The COVID-19 global pandemic shows how the competing interests of the major powers including the USA and China have paralyzed the WHO and prevented it from working for the betterment of the world. In the domain of GHG, the role of WHO becomes important. WHO works as an actor by creating rules, norms, codes of conduct and forum by being a meeting place for states and non-state actors on the issues related with a global health concern and work as a resource by serving as a facilitator of knowledge creation. Thus, promoting global health governance in general and its institutions, in particular, becomes crucial for ensuring health security globally.

Narratives on Global Health Governance: A Brief Account

In the nineteenth century, there were impressive advancements in the areas of transportation, telecommunications, international trade, and commerce. One can mention that in 1850, the volume of world shipping tonnage was 700,000 tons that increased to 26,200,000 tons in 1910. The expansion of international trade and commerce also resulted in the spread of diseases internationally (Harrison 2012). Preventing epidemic diseases was necessary for commercial purposes. It is worthy to note that the outbreaks of cholera, threats of yellow fever, bubonic plague, smallpox, and typhus contributed to the development of global cooperation on health and thus international health regulations (Clinton and Sridhar 2017). Between 1816 and 1899, six cholera pandemics (1816–26, 1829–51, 1852–60, 1863–75, 1881–96, 1899–1923) occurred which infected Asia, Europe, and the Middle East. Consequently, global initiatives to prevent diseases were also manifested, which can be identified as the early stage of global health governance. In 1851, the International Sanitary Conference, for instance, was held, which was followed by ten more conferences on health over the next 50 years (Zacher and Keefe 2008). It is argued that international cooperation on health was accelerated during the four International Sanitary Conferences of the 1890s (Zacher and Keefe 2008).

In 1903, twenty countries from Europe, North America, the Middle East, Latin America met in Paris, which resulted in an agreement on dealing with future outbreaks of cholera, plague, and yellow fever. Consequently, four years later, in 1907, the first international health agency called Office International d'hygiène Publique (OIHP), based in Paris, came into being (Clinton and Sridhar 2017). The scientific breakthrough on biomedical discoveries was imperative in the initiatives for such global health institutionalisation. After the establishment of the League of Nations in 1919, there were negotiations for establishing an international health organisation with a global scope not only addressing infectious diseases but also nutrition, safe water supplies, better housing and other health challenges as some constituents expected. Thus, in 1920, the League of Nation's Health Organisation (LNHO) came into being with a central focus on surveillance and control of epidemic diseases as they were mostly concerned by the wealthiest/developed states. One of the successful examples of the organisation was receiving surveillance reports from 140 port cities globally (Clinton and Sridhar 2017). In addition, LNHO slightly focused on non-infectious diseases, provided guidance on proper sanitation and made health systems recommendations, i.e., one doctor is required per 2,000 people. But as the donors' support declined significantly throughout the 1930s, it limited the LNHO's work particularly on non-infectious diseases. The LNHO also worked closely with China and Latin American states throughout the late 1920s and early 1930s emphasising on maternal and child health issues. In fact, international surveillance, monitoring, and reporting were significant areas of health cooperation following the First World War and up to the end of the Second World War (McInnes and Lee 2012:103). Liberal institutionalists argued that health should be a new pillar of post-war functionalism.

Until the end of the Second World War, international cooperation on health was stagnant. However, the end of the Second World War provided an impetus for an international health organisation to move the world forward. Thus, at the San Francisco Conference in 1945, the delegations of Brazil and China introduced a resolution for the calling of a special conference to establish an international health organisation. In February 1946, the United Nations organised an international conference in New York. The establishment of the World Health Organisation (WHO) in 1948 became a remarkable development in the history of contemporary GHG. The WHO has been identified as the centrepiece of global health governance. According to Article 1 of the WHO constitution, 'The objective of the World Health Organisation shall be the attainment by all peoples of the highest possible level of health'. Its mandate, i.e., 'to promote and protect the health of all peoples...without distinction of race, religion, political belief, economic or social condition' (Brundtland 2011:83). To understand the role of the WHO as a global health agency with regard to global health governance, one needs to mention the International Sanitary Regulations (ISR), which were adopted by the World Health Assembly in 1951. Another development was the adoption of International Health Regulations (IHR) in 1969, which replaced the earlier ISR. IHR obligated member-states to report any cases of cholera, plague, or yellow fever or any other infectious disease outbreak within their boundaries.

One of the notable successes of the WHO is the eradication of deadly smallpox that killed millions globally. It is worthy to note that both the USA and the Soviet Union cooperated in this initiative to eradicate smallpox. In fact, the Soviet Union sponsored the first global smallpox eradication resolution in 1958. The initiative received momentum in 1966 when the USA, along with other states, expanded their hand to eradicate smallpox within ten years. Under the leadership of the WHO, it was possible to eradicate smallpox by 1979 (Clinton and Sridhar 2017). Despite such success, there were increasing tensions between the 'vertical' approach, which mainly deals with the infectious diseases, and the 'horizontal' approach, which focuses on the strengthening the entire health system and basic care services so that in the long term, infectious disease can also be prevented. However, the bilateral donors were more interested in vertical interventions (Clinton and Sridhar 2017). In 1978, the WHO and UNICEF convened an international conference on primary healthcare in Alma-Ata (Soviet Union, current-day Kazakhstan) where all the member-states of the WHO attended and expressed 'the need for urgent action by all governments, all health and development workers, and the world community to protect and promote the health of all the people of the world' (WHO 1978). Notably, for the first time, healthcare challenges of the developing states were seriously examined in the conference. The conference resulted in the Alma-Ata Declaration where health was identified as a fundamental human right; the role of international cooperation was also emphasised in the conference. As the Declaration reads, 'All countries should cooperate in a spirit of partnership and service to ensure primary health care for all people since the attainment of health by people in any one country directly concerns and benefits every other country' (WHO 1978). The Declaration urged the developed states to provide financial and technical support to meet the primary healthcare challenges of the developing nations.

At the beginning of the 1980s, there was an upsurge in international health collaboration, especially against the Ebola, SARS, HIV/AIDS outbreaks, which was primarily coordinated by the World Health Organisation. It is also worth mentioning the Revised International Health Regulations (IHR) (2005), which requires states to report any potential public health emergency of international concern to the WHO. The IHR play a crucial role in global health governance by setting global norms and standards.

The WHO, which has been the conventional global health agency, has been replaced by the World Bank in 1990 as the largest funder of health. Though the World Bank began its functions as a pre-eminent development institution, it also took entry as a global health agency and eclipsed the functions of the WHO. In fact, the World Bank started direct lending for health in 1980. Within three years, it became the largest funders for health (World Bank 1988). The institution began influencing the world's health system. In this case, one needs to critically look at the policies of the Bank on the health systems of the developing countries. In 1987, the World Bank published an entire policy paper on health sector reforms in the developing countries, which provides four prescriptions for developing countries to reform their health systems: (i) Charging fees for government health services, (ii) Encouraging privatisation of healthcare services, (iii) Promoting private insurance programmes (companies), (iv) Decentralising the management of the public health system (World Bank 1988). In fact, these policies were linked with the World Bank's structural adjustment policy and were mandatory for the indebted countries to reform their healthcare system/policy (Maciocco and Italian Global Health Watch 2008). Maciocco and Italian Global Health Watch (2008:38) note that:

These four directives are strongly linked. The introduction of user fees in government structures is not only a way of making users pay, it is also essential for promoting insurance systems. On the other hand, without an insurance system the government hospitals cannot apply tariffs sufficient to cover costs. The privatisation of services and programme decentralisation are the other two essential components of the proposed strategy, clearly meant to reduce to a minimum the role of governments in health care, leaving space for systems of private care and health insurance. The effects of structural adjustment policies were soon rapidly and dramatically evident.

Since the publication of the World Bank policy document on health reform (1987), many developing countries were compelled to introduce fees for public healthcare services. In fact, the introduction of user fees for public healthcare services was a condition for loans and aid from international donors (Whitehead et al. 2001:833). In addition, people's out-of-pocket expenses increased drastically due to the increased privatisation of healthcare services. Thus, many families became poor due to the increased costs of healthcare services. This situation is defined as a 'medical poverty trap' (Whitehead et al. 2001:833). It is argued that among many negative consequences of World Bank policy, one needs to mention untreated morbidity, reduced access to care, long-term impoverishment, and irrational use of drugs (Whitehead et al. 2001). Since public health services are the only hope for millions of people in developing countries, World Bank policy on health reform had immense negative implications for the health security of those people. In fact, within the World Bank, health is seen as an economic commodity instead of a right. Ugalde and Jackson (1995:525) argue that 'the World Bank's approach to health fits its ideologically-driven development model which favours nations of the North at the expense of the poor of the South'. For Godlee (1997:1359), 'The moves towards privatisation and tertiary care are mirrored by reduced emphasis on and provision of primary and preventive care'. It is also worthy to note that the World Bank policy on health reform has increased health inequities and worsened access to healthcare for the world's most vulnerable people.

There is a resurgence of other non-state actors in global health governance. One also needs to look at the development of global public-private partnerships such as the Global Alliance for Vaccines and Immunisation (GAVI),* the Global Fund to fight AIDS, Tuberculosis and Malaria, private foundations, i.e., the Bill and Melinda Gates Foundation, civil society organisations in the global health governance. On a positive note, the GAVI Alliance has achieved substantial achievement in the domain of vaccines and immunisation. On the contrary, Global Fund (G.F.) has been very influential in shaping major international health policy. However, it is argued that

> No health system in the world is actually built on "vertical" programmes. Nonetheless because of the G.F. an unduly strict selective approach to health care delivery has often been introduced into poor countries in the early stages of their development; this has had destructive effects on their health systems, as even the IMF itself has been forced to admit (Maciocco and Italian Global Health Watch 2008:47).

Though many embrace the rise of a multitude of actors in global health governance, it has created impediments to the better functioning of global health governance since there is a fight over resource allocation. In this regard, it is argued that 'The multitude of actors involved in global health in recent decades has led to a problem of direction and competing interests fighting over finance. A multiplicity of actors bring a plurality of ideas but also dilute claims to the public nature of global health' (Harman 2014:664).

COVID-19 Global Pandemic: A Crisis of Global Health Governance

We see that global health governance failed in the case of the COVID-19 global pandemic when the world needed it most. In fact, one can argue that if global health governance would work properly in the case of the COVID-19 pandemic, the pandemic could have been prevented and controlled. In this chapter, we argue that global health governance failed as the norm of international cooperation did not work out, the crisis of global leadership, and the marginalisation of science from policy processes.

---

* Alliance between governments, UN agencies, the vaccine industry, private sector and civil society organizations.

Failure of the Norm of Cooperation

Norm is one of the key dimensions of global health governance. According to the WHO principle, 'The health of all peoples is fundamental to the attainment of peace and security and is dependent upon the fullest cooperation of individuals and States' (WHO 2006:1). Thus, the norm would be the 'fullest cooperation of individuals and States' during addressing the COVID-19 global pandemic. But, ironically, non-cooperation from many states, including the major powers, signals the violation of norms. The blame game, politics of denial, bypassing the role of the WHO, absence of concrete regional and international cooperation are evident in addressing the COVID-19 crisis. It is reported that by March 2020, 60 countries, including the European Union, restricted exporting medical equipment, i.e., personal protective equipment, including face shields, surgical masks and gowns (Boykoff 2020). By the first week of April 2020, the USA restricted export of critical medical gear (Bade 2020, Toosi 2020). Some countries, including the United Kingdom, banned exporting essential medicines for COVID-19 patients (Rees 2020).

A joint study by the European University Institute, Global Trade Alert, and World Bank Group (2020) finds that since the beginning of 2020, 86 jurisdictions were reported which executed a total of 157 export controls of medical supplies and medicines. Export curbs on food are also manifested (See Table 1). Notably, 27 jurisdictions are reported executing a total of 39 export controls since the beginning of 2020 (European University Institute et al. 2020).

Table 1: Total Number of New Export Controls and Import Reforms in Sensitive Sectors since January 2020, by Month (Updated on May 22, 2020)

Month of implementation	Number of new cases	Type	Sector
January	2	Export curb	Medical sector
February	16	Export curb	Medical sector
March	96	Export curb	Medical sector
April	41	Export curb	Medical sector
May	2	Export curb	Medical sector
February	1	Export curb	Food

(Contd.)

Month of implementation	Number of new cases	Type	Sector
March	16	Export curb	Food
April	22	Export curb	Food
January	3	Import reforms	Medical sector
February	5	Import reforms	Medical sector
March	84	Import reforms	Medical sector
April	56	Import reforms	Medical sector
May	5	Import reforms	Medical sector
January	1	Import reforms	Food
February	-	Import reforms	Food
March	10	Import reforms	Food
April	19	Import reforms	Food
May	2	Import reform	Food

Source: EUI et al. (2020).

Table 1 demonstrates that due to the coronavirus outbreak, there are many cases of export ban on medical supplies and medicine and on food, which signals the return of protectionism, and nationalism, which might be counterproductive primarily for global health governance. World Bank economists Michele Ruta and Aaditya Mattoo in their study found that just seven countries account for 70 per cent of ventilator exports. They estimated that if just one producer imposes an export ban, world prices would go up by 10 per cent. Ruta claimed that 'If more countries do it, the price increase would be much larger' (Boykoff 2020). Nahal Toosi (2020) writes that 'Developing countries...are terrified of being left behind in the race for personal protective equipment, or PPE, and other materials because they cannot match the purchasing power of the U.S. and other wealthy countries'.

The American policy of developing a vaccine 'only for U.S. citizens' (Manderson and Levine 2020) also demonstrates the non-cooperative attitude towards the rest of the world. The rise of 'national interest' in the case of addressing the COVID-19 crisis is ironic for the betterment of the world's people. It is also worthy to note that 'In Europe, walls were raised between countries for the first time in generations as the nation state re-emerged and the European Union seemed, for a time, a mere bystander' (Burns 2020).

MacDonald (2020) writes in *East Asia Forum* that the behaviour of the USA, China, Russia demonstrates 'their preference of self-interest over cooperation through international institutions. They view the pandemic not as a collective action challenge requiring the relaxation of strategic rivalry and tensions, but rather as a geopolitical battleground over power and position'. Rather than focusing on a coordinated approach to resolve the pandemic, global powers were more interested in spreading disinformation on who was responsible for the virus, from where it is originated, who is leading the fight against the virus, etc. It is also reported that China imposed restrictions on the origin of coronavirus research and publication (Gan et al. 2020). Such non-cooperative attitude by many, including the European and North American states, underscores the violation of the norm of cooperation, which is one of the defining features of global health governance. One can also argue that the non-cooperative attitude emerged due to the clear crisis of global leadership, which is explained in the next section.

Crisis of Global Leadership

Global health governance failed due to the crisis of global leadership. In fact, global leadership matters in the context of addressing global issues including health challenges as the self-interest and irresponsible behaviour of a few can pose dire consequences for the entire world (Chanda and Froetschel 2012). We argue that power politics or narrowly defined regime/national interest made the global leadership crisis in dealing with the COVID-19 global pandemic. Consequently, a coordinated global response is absent which allowed the virus to spread globally and increased the number of cases and fatalities. The Sino-U.S. rivalry primarily created the crisis of global leadership, which made international coordination difficult in dealing with COVID-19. In this regard, James Crabtree (2020) writes that 'geopolitical fissures, and strained relations between the USA and China in particular, have badly undermined early international efforts to respond to the coronavirus pandemic'. United Nations Secretary-General Antonio Guterres also lamented the lack of global leadership in the fight against coronavirus, as Reuters reports (Nichols 2020).

In fact, foreign ministers from G-7 member states held a meeting but failed to issue a joint statement on the subject of novel coronavirus as U.S. President Donald Trump insisted the member-states call the outbreak of coronavirus as a 'Wuhan virus' (Hudson and Mekhennet 2020). On the contrary, Chinese Foreign Ministry representative Zhao Lijian tweeted on March 12 that it 'might be U.S. Army who brought the epidemic to Wuhan' (quoted in Crabtree 2020). Concrete step from G-20 are absent in dealing with COVID-19.

In April 2020, the USA announced stopping of funding of WHO following its criticism that it was biased towards China and failed to address the coronavirus pandemic. On May 29, 2020, Donald Trump announced the cutting of ties with the WHO. According to Trump, 'Because they [WHO] have failed to make the requested and greatly needed reforms, we will be today terminating our relationship with the World Health Organisation and redirecting those funds to other worldwide and deserving urgent global public health needs' (quoted in Holland and Nichols 2020). Lawrence O. Gostin and Matthew M. Kavanagh write in the *Washington Post* (April 13, 2020) that Donald Trump's criticisms of the WHO in the case of coronavirus outbreak are wrong as the WHO took measures from the very beginning and the USA was well informed about the virus. They further write that:

> The U.S. failure to lead a coordinated response is sure to lengthen the duration of this pandemic. Weakening and defunding the WHO will undermine the global response—worsening the health and economic devastation to come in poorer countries. None of this will be good for Americans' health, the U.S. economy or the political survival of U.S. leaders.

Against the announcement of Trump, Donna McKay, executive director of Physicians for Human Rights, contends that 'It's important to remember that the WHO is a platform for cooperation among countries. Walking away from this critical institution in the midst of an historic pandemic will hurt people both in the United States and around the world' (quoted in Holland and Nichols 2020). Notably, the USA is the largest funder of the WHO. It provided 15 per cent of WHO's 2018-19 budget accounting more than US$ 400 million. According to Bill Gates, 'Halting funding for the World Health Organisation during a world health crisis is as dangerous as it sounds. The world needs the WHO now more than ever' (*BBC News*, April 15, 2020). Notably, the Bill & Melinda Gates Foundation is the second-largest funder of the WHO. In fact, the cut off of U.S. funding to international institutions that work on global public health is not new. In July 2002, the Bush Administration cut off all funding for the United Nations Population Fund that works on reproductive health and family planning on the 'false accusation' that UNFPA supported forced abortion and sterilisation in China (Ingram 2005). Notably, the USA was the largest funder of UNFPA.

In the past, it is seen that the USA claimed the international leadership in health by being the single largest donor of overseas development aid (ODA) for health (Ingram 2005). The USA led global responses to earthquakes, tsunamis, and the AIDS and Ebola crises which is absent in the case of COVID-19 (Gostin and Kavanagh 2020). In fact, one can claim that Donald Trump's indifference to multilateralism created barriers to global governance institutions including the WHO.

Marginalisation of the World Health Organisation
The World Health Organisation has traditionally been the leading international institution in global health governance. It has been advocating a global health agenda and working for the promotion and protection of global health since the beginning of its establishment. The institution also works to disseminate ideas, knowledge and best practices worldwide. The WHO plays an important role in shaping national health policies, especially in poor countries, and provides technical and operational assistance to the affected people/country/region, provides guidelines and recommendations about the types of treatments, and 'other similarly fundamental decisions that have had a substantial impact on the health conditions of a large number of people in need' (Chorev 2012:vii). Gro Harlem Brundtland, a former Director-General of WHO, notes (2011:83) that the WHO has played an important role in the reduction of child mortality rate by 60 per cent globally, smallpox and polio by 99

per cent. It is worthy to note that smallpox has killed more than 300 million people in the 20th century alone (Brundtland and Cousens 2020). The WHO has paved the way to increase the life expectancy and quality of life for millions around the world.

The WHO has been marginalised over the decades by the major powers considering their narrowly defined interests. For instance, the institution has remained underfunded for decades. Even calculating their specific interests, major powers/donors funded specific projects of the WHO. The current (2020) funding crisis of the WHO creates impediments for the smooth functioning in global health governance. Gostin (2017: 227) writes that WHO is financially and structurally weak, with a budget roughly one-quarter that of the CDC [Centers for Disease Control and Prevention, USA] and less than that of many large U.S. hospitals'. Kevin Rudd, a former Australian Prime Minister, claims that 'On any measure, the global response...on public health...has been unacceptably slow and disorganised' (quoted in Crabtree 2020).

The sudden cutting off of funding to the WHO in such a critical global health crisis, worsens human suffering around the world. While the USA announced a US$ 2.2 trillion coronavirus rescue package, the WHO faced an immediate funding gap of only US$ 20 million. According to the WHO Director-General Tedros Adhanom Ghebreyesus, 'To be very frank, if no new resources are received, we will run out of money before the end of the outbreak' (quoted in Usher 2020). Consequently, the WHO appealed directly for the first time in its history to the general public for financial support. By April 22, 2020, it had raised US$ 200 million which falls far short of the budget gap that the USA has widened. Thus, marginalisation of the WHO has been one of the major factors of the GHG crisis in the context of COVID-19.

Marginalisation of Science from Policy Processes

In Article 2 of the WHO constitution, it is mentioned that one of its functions would be 'to promote cooperation among scientific and professional groups which contribute to the advancement of health' (WHO 2006:2). In the case of global health governance, it is argued that 'Scientists and technical experts shape international public health norms and rules, and they compose much of the key staff at international health institutions' (Batniji and Songane 2014:65). Scientists and technical experts with similar interests and expertise are also called epistemic communities (Haas 1992). These epistemic communities play three key roles in policy-making, i.e., explaining the relationship between cause and effect, examining interlinkages between different issues, and framing, proposing, and identifying regulations (Haas 1992). In the case of global health governance, the role of the epistemic community is undeniable. But over the decades, science has been marginalised from health policy processes. The result is the helplessness of the world against the fight of the COVID-19 global pandemic and the devastating consequences.

Implications for South Asia

By April 1958, 1,300 people were dying each week in East Pakistan due to the outbreaks of smallpox and cholera which began in October 1957. In the first six months of 1958; 44,736 cholera cases were recorded which resulted in 20,444 deaths (Cockburn 1960:26). On the contrary, there were 10,438 cholera cases which caused 6,684 deaths. East Pakistan's public health sector was facing an acute shortage of money, doctors, and medical equipment due to the long-standing exploitation (economic, political, administrative, etc.) by West Pakistan. It is worthy to note that in April 1958, while East Pakistan was facing severe challenges to face these epidemics, regional and international cooperation was noticeable. Under the leadership of the WHO, twenty-one nations, and several voluntary agencies sent East Pakistan a total of 8,243,000 cc. of dry vaccine and 18,284,025 cc. of lymph vaccine to treat smallpox, and 2,475,600 cc. of vaccine to treat cholera. Five international teams came forward to give epidemiological assistance, including a team of 20 members from Afghanistan. This is how South Asian states were benefitting from global cooperation on health. In fact, it is worth mentioning that the first regional office for WHO was in the South-East, the Asia Region established in New Delhi in November 1948 which also underscores the significance of South-East Asia in the global health landscape. In fact, for the newly independent states, the South Asian health picture was bleak in the beginning. Dr. V.T.H. Gunaratne, the then regional director for WHO's South-East Asia Region, recalls the 25th anniversary of the World Health Organisation for South-East Asia, and remembers that:

> It is sometimes difficult to recall what conditions were like in 1947. Malaria was rampant. India alone had some 75 million cases of malaria, causing some 800,000 deaths a year. Some 2.5 million cases of tuberculosis led to half a million deaths annually. The situation was equally grim in other countries. Smallpox reigned unchecked, scarring, blinding and killing thousands. Plague and other common communicable diseases were ever-present menaces. In most of the newly independent countries, doctors and nurses were particularly scarce, and there were extremely limited facilities for training and preparing them. Finally, many countries were still attempting to deal with their health problems on a day-to-day basis, and there was a dearth of overall planning, often an absence of rational goals, and little attempt to improve training techniques (quoted in WHO 2018:6).

The above Quotation of Gunaratne demonstrates the health challenges of South Asia in the 1950s. Ninety per cent of the world's smallpox cases were found in WHO's South-East Asia Region. And due to the efforts of the WHO, smallpox has been eradicated from the world which was a major health challenge for the South Asian countries. Thus, South Asian countries have immensely benefitted from global health governance (See Tables 2 and 3).

Table 2: Reduction of Malaria Incidence in South Asia in the First Two Decades of WHO (Incidence of malaria per 100,000 population)

Country	Incidence (year)	Incidence (year)
Bangladesh	4,400 (1956)	5 (1965)
India	23,000 (1947)	13 (1961)
Maldives	40,000 (1964)	227 (1974)
Nepal	5,000 (1950)	44 (1968)
Sri Lanka	38,000 (1945)	0.2 (1963)

Source: WHO (2018:48).

Table 2 demonstrates that the incidence of malaria in South Asian countries has been reduced significantly because the WHO played a crucial role. South Asia received substantial importance in the domain of global health cooperation. In 1961, the Fourteenth World Health Assembly was held in New Delhi, India which was the first of its kind in Asia. Notably, delegates from 105 countries attended the opening session on 7 February. In the Assembly, the health challenges of developing countries, i.e., smallpox, infant mortality rate, yaws were critically discussed. Dr. V.T.H. Gunaratne, a former regional director of WHO's South-East Asia Region, contends that 'A serious obstacle...in providing health services...is the shortage of trained health manpower. Therefore, WHO is giving high priority to develop education and training programmes so that the Member-States will be in a position to prepare professional and auxiliary personnel in adequate numbers' (quoted in WHO 2018:69). Therefore, in 1972, the WHO established a regional teacher's training centre in Sri Lanka for human resource development in the health services of the region. Box 1 explains the health challenges of South Asia in the 1990s.

Box 1: South Asia in The State of the World's Children 1989

South Asia still contains the majority of the world's absolute poor, and most of its children are being born into communities where illiteracy, preventable diseases, poor growth, and early death are still common. More than one third of all the world's child deaths, for example, occur in just three South Asian countries—Bangladesh, India, and Pakistan. Vaccine-preventable diseases still kill over 1.5 million children every year in the seven SAARC countries. Approximately 85,000 more are disabled every year by polio. But recent progress has been rapid. Latest official figures show that the percentage of one-year-olds receiving all three shots of DPT vaccine is approximately 80 % in Sri Lanka, over 60 % in Pakistan, and almost 60 % in India. Lagging behind are Nepal (38%), Bhutan (16%), and Bangladesh (9%).

In all seven nations, diarrhoeal diseases are one of the most important causes of child death and child malnutrition, claiming more than 1.5 million young lives a year. (Source: UNICEF 1989: 26).

Box 1 shows that South Asia faced enormous health challenges over the decades. As chapter 2 in this book shows, the health security of the South Asian people in some parameters has improved. In that context, the role of global health governance needs to be acknowledged. For instance, the immunisation programmes run by the WHO have benefitted tens of thousands of poor, marginal people in South Asia. The Alma-Ata Declaration of WHO was immensely beneficial for the developing countries, including South Asian countries. The regional initiatives of the WHO have been imperative to eliminate measles, malaria, polio in some/all countries of South Asia (Table 3).

Table 3: Key WHO Success in the Elimination of Diseases in South Asia

Countries/Region	Elimination of Diseases
Bhutan, Maldives	Measles
Sri Lanka, Maldives	Malaria
India	Yaws-free
Maldives, Sri Lanka	Lymphatic Filariasis
South Asia	Maternal, neonatal tetanus elimination
South Asia	Polio free status
South Asia	Records world-beating gains in maternal, under-five, neonatal mortality

Source: WHO (2017).

In addition, the WHO publishes annual health statistics of its individual member-states on its official website to motivate South Asian states to uplift their health status. In the case of COVID-19, the guidelines and directions of the WHO were crucial for the South Asian countries to contain the spread of the disease. Thus, the marginalisation or failure of the global health governance institution, i.e., the WHO, will bring disastrous consequences for South Asian health security.

Looking Ahead

Passivity, lack of interest and splits in the global responses in the fight against COVID-19 signal a sorrow picture for global health governance in the post-COVID-19 era. As the earlier sections illustrate, the return of strong nationalism, protectionism in the COVID-19 period, might be counterproductive in the post-COVID-19 global health governance. Thus, the role of the WHO, international cooperation, global leadership, and science needs to be taken into consideration seriously by the states and non-state actors of the world for effective global health governance.

Prioritising Health

COVID-19 demonstrates that health issues need to be prioritised at the national, regional, and global level. In October 2019, the Nuclear Threat Initiative (NTI), and the Johns Hopkins Centre for Health Security jointly published the Global Health Security (GHS) Index 2019 which stated that none of the 195 countries, that make up the States/Parties to the 2005 International Health Regulations (IHR) is fully prepared to face a pandemic (NTI and the Johns Hopkins Centre for Health Security 2019). This shows that the states of the world are not serious enough about health challenges. The report also found that collectively, international preparedness to face a global pandemic is weak while Beth Cameron, vice president for global biological policy and programmes at the Nuclear Threat Initiative, contends that 'Health security is a collective responsibility' (cited in Sun 2019). Thus, health issues need to be prioritised for the benefit of all.

Promoting International Cooperation and Innovations

International cooperation becomes crucial to address infectious diseases. In favour of international cooperation on health, it is argued that 'citizens and politicians must be convinced that international cooperation for health has more than moral value: it is in everyone's self-interest' (Holloway 2015:1). In the case of the COVID-19 global pandemic, as explained in the above sections, the apparent absence of international cooperation made the crisis worse. In fact, the rise of protectionism, populism, and crisis of global leadership underscore the importance of international cooperation to face health challenges. As discussed earlier, even during the Cold War period, the WHO was able to achieve many successes in addressing the world's health challenges as the major powers cooperated on health issues. Eleanor Krassen Covan, in an editorial in *Health Care for Women International*, writes that 'Other viral issues will surely emerge if we don't find a way to work together' (Covan 2020:239). In the post-COVID-19 global health governance, international cooperation will be crucial as infectious diseases do not respect international borders, major powers' rivalry will disrupt global health governance severely which will affect everyone, protectionism will affect global health governance, and healthy nations will bring benefits to everyone. Thus, instead of narrowly defined national interest, the states of the world need to work together in promoting their common interest for the benefit of all on earth. International cooperation will be the key. In this context, the role of building global networks between scholars, scientists, and policymakers becomes imperative.

It is also important to promote innovations in global health governance. In this regard, G.H. Brundtland (2011:84), a former Director-General of WHO, writes that 'we must learn from recent innovations in global health, stretch and use them to their fullest potential, and identify new models that will further improve the efficiency and effectiveness of global health policy'.

Strengthening the Role of WHO

In the earlier sections, it was manifested that the role of the WHO has been marginalised and bypassed in addressing the COVID-19 global pandemic. The USA tried to paralyse the institution, which might be counterproductive for everyone in the long term. The world cannot afford to paralyse the only global institution that solely works on global health/public health. In fact, in this age of emerging and re-emerging infectious diseases, the developing world badly needs the help of the WHO. In the post-COVID-19 era, the role of the WHO needs to be reinvigorated. It is essential to reinforce whole health systems, instead of basing strategies on vertical programmes of the WHO.

Role of the Rising Powers

Against the absence of cooperation from the major powers in the issue of coronavirus, Adam P. MacDonald of Dalhousie University, emphasises the role of the smaller states 'to stabilise the global order' (MacDonald 2020). In fact, while the major powers closed their doors, countries like

Bangladesh and Vietnam expanded their helping hand. Bangladesh exported 6.5 million personal protective equipment (PPE) to the USA in May 2020 (*Samakal*, May 25, 2020). In the absence of U.S. leadership, the rising powers, i.e., China, India, Brazil, the E.U. need to come forward to fill the gap. There is a substantial increase in China's participation in global health governance (Chan 2011). Notably, China currently contributes more than 12 per cent of the U.N. budget which needs to be increased to fill the vacuum created by the USA.

Role of Epistemic Communities: Bring Science and Scientists Back in Policy Processes

One can argue that the role of scholars and scholarship would be necessary for better global health governance as a better theory (knowledge) translates into better policies. Instead of promoting extreme nationalism or populism, global governance institutions, including the WHO, international cooperation, regional cooperation needs to be embraced. In this regard, the role of the epistemic community would be essential. In fact, informed decision-making based on science becomes vital to deal with global health challenges, including pandemics. But COVID-19 shows the world that science cannot be neglected any more in the policy domain. The world might experience more health challenging infectious diseases in the coming decades, which require more investments in medical science. Thus, policymakers need to acknowledge the role of science and collaborate with natural and social science scientists.

Rethinking Contemporary World Politics

Hans J. Morgenthau claimed that international politics is nothing but 'power politics'. Though this power politics has defined the discourse of world politics over the decades, it becomes helpless in the face of diseases like COVID-19. COVID-19 has shown that even the most powerful countries in the world become defenceless. This power politics did not work for the vast majority of the people in the world, as demonstrated in the COVID-19 global crisis. We also see that the present world order, led by the economic globalisation (based on the principle of 'profit over people') has been imperative to make the present global health crisis as it made health a neglected issue area. Additionally, the neo-liberal economic model has created vast inequalities in societies. Deborah Hardoon finds that the incomes of the poorest 10 per cent of people increased by less than $ 3 a year between 1988 and 2011, while the incomes of the richest 1 per cent increased 182 times as much. Here, elites in society have access to health care. Health inequity is not a one-day outcome; rather, it is the outcome of the negative consequences of decades of world politics. It is argued that 'more than 30,000 children die daily from easily preventable diseases. The children who are hungry, homeless, and helpless; are not hungry, homeless, and helpless because it is their fault, or because it is natural: they are as they are because they are made to be hungry, homeless, and helpless. Global poverty is not an existential condition; it is the outcome of world politics—of human choices made in specific conditions' (Booth, 2007: 14-15). Thus, one can argue that the COVID-19 crisis is not a one-day outcome. Instead, it is the consequence of the long-standing narrowly defined world politics of the major powers.

The state is seen as the central unit of analysis in world politics. So, people's suffering and well-being are hardly taken into account in the discourse of world politics which needs to be problematised. One can argue that if global health were a priority area of world politics, this COVID-19 crisis could have been managed more efficiently within the shortest possible time, with fewer casualties/fatalities. COVID-19 has shown that the world has become reluctant to invest more in medical science compared to armaments. Thus, the contemporary world politics of by the powerful, of the powerful, and for the powerful, needs to be problematised. And people's well-being needs to be at the centre of world politics rather than the interests of the regimes, TNCs, lobby groups, and aristocrats. In this case, the study and practice of world politics needs to be re-designed/restructured. Thus, the world needs progressive politics. As the Commission on Social Determinants of Health (2008: 1) notes:

> The poor health of the poor, ...and the marked health inequities between countries are caused by the unequal distribution of power, income, goods, and services, globally and nationally. This unequal distribution of health-damaging experiences is in no sense a 'natural' phenomenon

but is the result of a toxic combination of poor social policies and programmes, unfair economic arrangements, and bad politics (cited in Schrecker and Bambra 2015:6).

It is argued that 'Politics, not just scientific discovery...remains the key challenge for global health governance' (Harman 2014:665). Therefore, this chapter strongly suggests that world politics needs to be redefined, safeguarding the welfare and well-being of the people. One cannot expect better global health governance if world politics is not fixed.

Conclusion

The COVID-19 global pandemic showed that people died, starved, protested, and cried for food, medicare in different corners of the world due to the impacts of the pandemic. The world has also witnessed a mother committing suicide as she failed to feed her children due to the lockdown measures. Tens of thousands of people were not able to buy food or medicine, to pay house rent and were thus suffering from hunger, disease, and anxieties. We have also seen that nurses were protesting in front of the White House demanding PPE (personal protection equipment). It is quite ironic that the superpower spends billions of dollars on armaments but is not able to provide PPE to address the pandemic. The sufferings of the people worsened as global health governance failed due to non-cooperation from the major powers, the crisis of global leadership, the marginalisation of the WHO and science from policy processes.

This chapter finds that in the post-COVID-19 era, the picture of global health governance would be disastrous if power politics dominates in the decision-making processes. The WHO, which provides equal opportunity to every state in the world by one country/one vote in the World Health Assembly, has been paralysed by the major powers. In fact, the states of the world, especially the developing world, cannot afford to lose support from the WHO as it is the only inter-governmental organisation that works on global health protection and promotion. More specifically, South Asia will be severely affected if the sole global health governance institution, i.e., the World Health Organisation, fails. For better global health governance, the World Health Organisation needs to be strengthened with financial strength, legal, and enforcement power. In fact, the world needs to be well-prepared for the next outbreak.

In the post-COVID-19 era, the rivalry between the major powers will worsen the global health crisis, which will affect everyone, especially the people in developing countries. Or one can argue that competition will make everyone vulnerable to future global health crises. Thus, in this rapidly changing and interconnected world, there is no alternative to promote global health governance based on international cooperation instead of rivalry.

REFERENCES

Bade, G. (2020, April 3). Despite expanded DPA, confusion reigns over coronavirus industrial response. *Politico*. Retrieved from https://www.politico.com/news/2020/04/03/trump-dpa-medical-goods-164036

Batniji, R. Songane, F. (2014). Contemporary global health governance: Origins, functions, and challenges. In G.W. Brown, G. Yamey, and S. Wamala (Eds.), *The handbook of global health policy*, (pp. 63-76), John Wiley & Sons, Ltd.

BBC News, (2020, April 15). Coronavirus: U.S. to halt funding to WHO, says Trump. Retrieved from https://www.bbc.com/news/world-us-canada-52289056

Booth, K. (2007). *Theory of world security*, New York: Cambridge University Press.

Boykoff, P. (2020, March 28). In the race to secure medical supplies, countries ban or restrict exports. *CNN*. Retrieved from https://edition.cnn.com/2020/03/27/business/medical-supplies-export-ban/index.html

Brundtland, G. H. (2011). U.N. efforts for global health: Instituting innovations for improvement. *Harvard International Review*, 33 (1), 83-87.

Brundtland, G. H., Cousens, E. (2020, June 4). World leaders must fund a COVID-19 vaccine plan before it's too late for millions. *The Guardian*. Retrieved from https://www.theguardian.com/commentisfree/2020/jun/04/world-leaders-fund-COVID-19-vaccine-global-vaccine-summit

Burns, N. (2020, May 15). GWU commencement address delivered on May 15, 2020. Belfer Centre for Science and International Affairs. Harvard University. Retrieved from https://www.belfercenter.org/publication/gwu-commencement-address-delivered-may-15-2020

Chan, L. (2011). *China engages global health governance: Responsible stakeholder or system-transformer?*. New York: Palgrave Macmillan.

Chorev, N. (2012). *The World Health Organization between north and south*. New York: Cornell University Press.

Clinton, C. & Sridhar, D. (2017). *Governing Global Health: Who runs the world and why?*. New York: Oxford University Press.

Cockburn, T.A. (1960). Epidemic crisis in East Pakistan April-July, 1958. *Public Health Reports (1896-1970)*. 75 (1), 26-36.

Commission on Global Governance (1995). *Our global neighbourhood*, Oxford: Oxford University Press.

Covan, E.K. (2020). COVID-19 uncertainty. *Health Care for Women International*, 41(3), 239-239.

Crabtree, J. (2020, April 15). How coronavirus exposed the collapse of global leadership. *Nikkei Asian Review*. Retrieved from https://asia.nikkei.com/Spotlight/Cover-Story/How-coronavirus-exposed-the-collapse-of-global-leadership

Dodgson, R., Lee, K. & Drager, N. (2002). Global health governance: A conceptual review. Discussion Paper Number 1. Geneva: WHO.

European University Institute, Global Trade Alert, and World Bank Group (2020). The COVID-19 pandemic: 21st century approaches to tracking trade policy responses in-real time. Retrieved from https://www.globaltradealert.org/reports/54

Gan, N., Hu, C. & Watson, I. (2020, April 16). Beijing tightens grip over coronavirus research, amid US-China row on virus origin. *CNN*. Retrieved from https://edition.cnn.com/2020/04/12/asia/china-coronavirus-research-restrictions-intl-hnk/index.html

Godlee, F. (1997). WHO reform and global health: Radical restructuring is the only way ahead. *BMJ: British Medical Journal*. 314 (7091), 1359-1360.

Gostin, L. O. (2017). 'America first': Prospects for global health. *The Milbank Quarterly*, 95 (2), 224-228.

Gostin, L.O. & Kavanagh, M.M. (2020, April 13). Why Trump and his allies' criticisms of the WHO are wrong. *The Washington Post*. Retrieved from https://www.msn.com/en-gb/news/coronavirus/opinions-why-trump-and-his-allies-criticisms-of-the-who-are-wrong/ar-BB12AhT6

Haas, P. M. (1992). Introduction: Epistemic communities and international policy coordination. *International Organization*. 46(1), 1–35.

Hardoon, D., Ayele, S., and Fuentes-Nieva, R. (2016). An economy for the 1%, 210 Oxfam Briefing Paper, Oxford: Oxfam International.

Harman, S. (2014). Global health governance. In T. G. Weiss & R. Wilkinson (Eds.), *International organisation and global governance* (p. 656-667). Abingdon, Oxon and New York: Routledge.

Harrison, M. (2012). *Contagion: How commerce has spread disease*. New Haven and London: Yale University Press.

Holland, S. & Nichols, M. (2020, May 30). Trump cutting U.S. ties with World Health Organization over virus. *Reuters*. Retrieved from https://www.reuters.com/article/us-health-coronavirus-trump-who/trump-cutting-us-ties-with-world-health-organization-over-virus-idUSKBN2352YJ

Holloway, D. T. (2015). Self-interest as motivation for international cooperation toward universal healthcare. *Harvard Public Health Review*, 5, 1-5.

Hudson, J. & Mekhennet, S. (2020, March 26). G-7 failed to agree on statement after U.S. insisted on calling coronavirus outbreak 'Wuhan virus'. *Washington Post*. Retrieved from https://www.washingtonpost.com/national-security/g-7-failed-to-agree-on-statement-after-us-insisted-on-calling-coronavirus-outbreak-wuhan-virus/2020/03/25/f2bc7a02-6ed3-11ea-96a0-df4c5d9284af_story.html

Ingram, A. (2005). Global leadership and global health: Contending meta-narratives, divergent responses, fatal consequences. *International Relations*. 19(4), 381–402.

Maciocco, G., Italian Global Health Watch (2008). From Alma-Ata to the Global Fund: The History of International Health Policy. *Social Medicine*, 3 (1), 36-48.

MacDonald, A.P. (2020, April 16). Power politics threatens global cooperation to combat COVID-19. *East Asia Forum*. Retrieved from https://www.eastasiaforum.org/

2020/04/16/power-politics-threatens-global-cooperation-to-combat-COVID-19/

Manderson, L., & Levine, S. (2020). COVID-19, risk, fear, and fallout. *Medical Anthropology*. DOI: 10.1080/01459740.2020.1746301

McInnes, C. & Lee, K. (2012). *Global health and international relations*. Cambridge, UK: Polity.

McInnes, C., Kamradt-Scott, A., Lee, K., Roemer-Mahler, A., Rushton, S. & Williams, O. W. (2014). *The transformation of global health governance*. Hampshire: Palgrave Macmillan.

Nichols, M. (2020, May 1). U.N. chief laments lack of global leadership in coronavirus fight. Reuters. Retrieved from https://www.reuters.com/article/us-health-coronavirus-guterres/u-n-chief-laments-lack-of-global-leadership-in-coronavirus-fight-idUSKBN22C3IS

NTI and the Johns Hopkins Centre for Health Security (2019). Global Health Security Index: Building Collective Action and Accountability. Retrieved from https://www.ghsindex.org/wp-content/uploads/2020/04/2019-Global-Health-Security-Index.pdf

Rees, V. (2020, March 23). U.K. bans parallel exporting of crucial medicines to help COVID-19 patients. European *Pharmaceutical Review*. Retrieved from https://www.europeanpharmaceuticalreview.com/news/115637/uk-bans-parallel-exporting-of-crucial-medicines-to-help-COVID-19-patients/

Samakal. (2020, May 25). Beximco exported 6.5 million PPE to the United States [In Bangla]. Retrieved from https://samakal.com/economics-others/article/200524289/%E0%A7%AC%E0%A7%AB-%E0%A6%B2%E0%A6%BE%E0%A6%96%20E0%A6%AA%E0%A6%BF%E0%A6%AA%E0%A6%BF%E0%A6%87-%E0%A6%97%E0%A6%BE%E0%A6%89%E0%A6%A8-%E0%A6%B0%E0%A6%AA%E0%A7%8D%E0%A6%A4%E0%A6%BE%E0%A6%A8%E0%A6%BF%E0%A6%AC%E0%A7%87%E0%A6%95%E0%A7%8D%E0%A6%B8%E0%A6%BF%E0%A6%AE%E0%A6%95%E0%A7%8B%E0%A6%B0

Schrecker, T. & Bambra, C. (2015). *How politics makes us sick: Neoliberal epidemics*. Hampshire and New York: Palgrave McMillan.

Sun, L. H. (2019, October 24). None of these 195 countries — the U.S. included — is fully prepared for a pandemic, report says. *The Washington Post*. Retrieved from https://www.washingtonpost.com/health/2019/10/24/none-these-countries-us-included-is-fully-prepared-pandemic-report-says/

Toosi, N. (2020, April 3). 'Lord of the Flies: PPE Edition': U.S. cast as culprit in global scrum over coronavirus supplies. *Politico*. Retrieved from https://www.politico.com/news/2020/04/03/ppe-world-supplies-coronavirus-163955

Ugalde, A. & Jackson, J. T. (1995). The World Bank and international health policy: A critical review. *Journal of International Development*. 7 (3), 525-541.

UNICEF (1989). *The State of the World's Children, 1989*. Walton Street, Oxford: Oxford University Press.

Usher, A. D. (2020, March 28). WHO launches crowdfund for COVID-19 response. *The Lancet*. Retrieved from https://www.thelancet.com/journals/lancet/article/PIIS0140-6736(20)30719-4/fulltext

Whitehead, M., Dahlgren, G. & Evans, T. (2001). Equity and health sector reforms: can low-income countries escape the medical poverty trap? *Lancet*. 358: 833–36.

WHO (1978, September 12). Declaration of Alma-Ata. International Conference on Primary Health Care, Alma-Ata, USSR, 6-12 September. Retrieved from http://www.who.int/publications/almaata_declaration_en.pdf

WHO (2006, October). Constitution of the World Health Organization. *Basic Documents*, Forty-fifth edition, Supplement.

WHO (2017). *From vision to results: Advancing health for billions in the South-East Asia Region.* New Delhi: World Health Organization, Regional Office for South-East Asia. Licence: CC BY-NC-SA 3.0 IGO.

WHO (2018). *A healthier South-East Asia: 70 years of WHO in the region.* New Delhi. World Health Organization, Regional Office for South-East Asia. Licence: CC BY-NC-SA 3.0 IGO.

World Bank (1988). Financing health services in developing countries: An agenda for reform (English). A World Bank policy study. Washington DC: World Bank. Retrieved from http://documents.worldbank.org/curated/en/468091468137379607/Financing-health-services-in-developing-countries-an-agenda-for-reform

Zacher, M.W. & Keefe, T.J. (2008). *The politics of global health governance: United by contagion.* New York: Palgrave Macmillan.

8

Conclusion: Way Forward

The novel coronavirus disease or COVID-19 has shattered everyone in the world with varying degrees and scale. It created human insecurity for millions and millions of people in the world, including in South Asia. Whether weak or powerful, poor or rich, capitalist or socialist, every state in the world has been affected by this global pandemic. It will be written as a black chapter in human history that will never be forgotten. As mentioned in chapter one, the world has never experienced such a challenging event after the Second World War. Against this backdrop, this book has investigated the human security implications of COVID-19 for South Asia. In the domain of human security, the subjects of health security, food security, economic security, and environmental security have been primarily covered. Two other linking chapters, i.e., the chapters on the role of regional cooperation and global health governance help to understand how the region and the world have responded to the challenge of the global pandemic and how they can respond more efficiently and effectively to any future pandemic. This concluding chapter focuses on policy imperatives. However, the following way forward can be taken into consideration by the academic and policy community in South Asia and beyond.

First, human security in South Asia, both in policy and scholarship, which has been neglected over the decades, needs to be mainstreamed. One of the sources of abundance for South Asia is its population. Thus, it becomes important to invest in South Asian people. In this context, in the policy domain, human security needs to be promoted in South Asia, taking the human as the referent object of security. Instead of national security, human security needs to be prioritised in the region, taking lessons from the COVID-19 global pandemic. As chapter two on health security shows, the issue of health security in South Asia has been a neglected area, both in policy and scholarship, over the decades due to the dominance of military security and the politicisation of security. Thus, COVID-19 shows how poor and fractured the healthcare system in South Asia is. Due to the weak healthcare sector, the poor and the marginal sections in society become most vulnerable to health challenges. Therefore, this book strongly suggests that South Asia's broken healthcare infrastructure needs to be reinvigorated. In this case, health needs to be the top-most priority for the region. Consequently, a unified-region wide strategy for preparedness and response will be imperative to face any future pandemic/epidemic. Infection prevention and control, disease surveillance also become important which requires generous investments in health.

In the case of scholarship, there is a paucity of human security research in South Asia. Thus, it becomes important to promote human security scholarship in the region. In this context, introducing human security courses in South Asia at the undergraduate and graduate levels in the discipline of International Relations and Political Science becomes essential. There is a clear need to promote collaborative research and insights on human security issues. Thus, South Asian states need to collaborate on joint research on health and other human security issues, both from natural and social science perspectives.

Second, in chapter three, it is found that COVID-19 has been a critical source of food insecurity for millions of poor and marginal people in South Asia. More specifically, food availability, accessibility, nutrition access and utilisation have been severely affected due to the impacts of the pandemic. To address food insecurity in South Asia, there is no alternative but to prioritise agriculture at the national and regional levels and save the farmers. As found in chapter seven, many countries restricted exporting food items due to the COVID-19 outbreak. In addition, there is also a signal for the return of strong nationalism and a protectionist policy that would be counterproductive to future food security for many countries in the world. Thus, states in South Asia and beyond need to stabilise the food system and keep trade open to achieve a win-win situation. South Asian countries need to focus on deepening regional agriculture cooperation and remove tariffs and non-tariff barriers and simplify customs clearance procedures for imports of agricultural products, essential drugs and equipment. Specifically, the negative list of agro-products needs to be addressed.

Third, addressing the economic insecurities (created from COVID-19 and beyond) of the people in South Asia becomes important as chapter four reveals. The growing inequalities in societies need to be addressed by ensuring minimum living standards and social protective policies. In this case, a strong economy will be imperative to provide resources in the human security sectors, including health security. Regional economic cooperation based on efficient and equitable trade practices becomes essential for building strong economies nationally. There is also a clear need for a fair distribution of the dividends of growth. Finally, it is reiterated that without due attention to the sources of economic insecurity in South Asia, no sustainable progress will be achieved.

Fourth, it becomes important to deepen cooperation on preserving the environment, both at the regional and global levels, to ensure the environmental security of the people in South Asia and beyond. Air pollution and climate change have been key sources of environmental insecurity for millions of people in South Asia and globally. In chapter five, it is demonstrated that COVID-19 has been a blessing for the global environment, particularly in the case of air pollution and global climate change due to the reduction of pollutants and carbon emission. It becomes important to take a lesson from COVID-19 and maintain a healthy balance between corporate profits and the environment for the enhancement of environmental security in South Asia and beyond. In this case, focusing on an environmentally sensitive climate policy, promoting renewable energy and other low-carbon sources, reinforcing regional initiatives, and ending the North-South divide in global environmental politics and reducing emissions become essential.

Fifth, as chapters six and seven find, regional and global cooperation is needed to face any future infectious disease. In this book, it is found that the narrowly defined national interest, restrictive trade policy, return of protectionism in the case of critical medical supplies or food supplies worsened the global health crisis against the fight to contain COVID-19. Thus, a concerted regional effort is needed to ensure the human security of the people in the region, which requires deepening regional cooperation. From a global perspective, there is no alternative to promotion of international cooperation on health. It is also suggested that developed countries need to expand technical, financial and logistic support as well as capacity building for the developing countries.

Sixth, it becomes necessary to prioritise health on the global agenda. In fact, recent outbreaks of Ebola, Zika, bird flu, and novel coronavirus underscore the necessity of prioritising health in the global agenda which often becomes marginalised due to the predominance of hard security/ or high political issues. The people in developing countries are mostly vulnerable to the impacts of infectious diseases considering the lack of improved healthcare systems, lack of cooperation at the global level and the failure of global health governance as COVID-19 has shown. World politics, based on the realist paradigm, which does not work for the vast majority of people, needs to be problematised. In this multidimensional, interdependent world, health challenges easily travel across borders and this makes states and non-states vulnerable to infectious diseases. Thus, the global health agency, i.e., the World Health Organisation, needs to be strengthened instead of marginalising it. The manner in which the WHO was bypassed/marginalised in the case of the COVID-19 global pandemic is pathetic. It is the developing world that will be mostly vulnerable in the absence of a strong WHO. In the case of prioritising health in the global agenda, along with strengthening the WHO, the crisis of global leadership, as shown in the case of COVID-19, needs to be addressed. In this case, the role of the middle powers, and emerging powers, i.e. China, India, Brazil, India, Japan, and the European Union needs to be pushed forward to fix the vulnerable world health system for the benefit of all as the chapter six argues.

Seventh, should South Asia deepen cooperation with China? The South Asian economy is closely linked with China's. Though one can witness some rivalries at the political level between India and China and between the USA and China, they maintain good economic relations except for some rhetoric. In fact, in the light of the COVID-19 global pandemic, South Asia might be affected by the changing geopolitics in the world arena, especially in the case of US-China rivalry. It is noticed that while many countries were closing their windows of cooperation, India and China came forward to help out South Asian countries with medical equipment though there was criticism of their objectives. Therefore, it is suggested that instead of nurturing rivalries, if South Asian countries could deepen their cooperation with China based on a 'win-win situation', it would bring positive outcomes for the people of the region in the context of securing and sustaining human security.

To conclude, South Asia is a rising region with immense potential. As chapter six shows, the region has more potential in terms of demography and social resilience. In the pre-COVID-19 world, it was predicted that the twenty-first century would be the Asian century where South Asia would play an important role. In fact, the rise of Bangladesh, India and Sri Lanka is well recognised by both the policy and academic communities. Thus, in the post-COVID-19 world, South Asian countries need to come together to face the consequences of the pandemic and to be back on the right track. In this case, the role of the leadership, epistemic community, and other civil society actors would be necessary. Considering its geography, economic and military capabilities, and the multidimensional relations with its neighbouring countries, India needs to play a constructive role to raise the region and thus, South Asian regionalism, for the well-being of the people in the region.

With regard to the contributions of this study, it can be claimed that this book will fill the existing knowledge gap in the COVID-19 and human security literature in South Asia. The findings and the policy imperatives of the study would be necessary for South Asian policy makers to reframe their policies and move the region forward. With regard to future research agenda, one can investigate COVID-19 implications in other human security areas, i.e., personal security, political security and community security in South Asia.

*

Index

Abdullah, 18
Abramowitz, Jonathan S., 32
Adlakha, Nidhi, 100
Afghanistan, 16-19, 22, 43, 48, 52-53, 55, 70-71, 73, 97, 105
Afghanistan-Pakistan border, 54
Agriculture, 49, 55
Ahmed, Mahfuz, 100
AIDS epidemic, 15
AIIB, 57
Air Pollution, 96-98, 103-5, 108, 110, 112, 115, 176
Air Traffic, 94
Al Jazeera, 17, 22, 96, 100, 109
Aldis, William, 13
Allenby, Braden R., 95
Alma-Ata Declaration, 151, 164
Almond, Douglas, 3
Amb Nicholas Burns, 146
Anadolu Agency, 49, 50
Ananda Bazar Patrika, 24
Annan, Kofi, UN Secretary-General, 6
ASEAN Regional Forum (ARF), 128, 131
Asia Pacific Economic Cooperation (APEC), 130
Asian Development Bank (ADB), 79
Association of Southeast Asian Nations (ASEAN), 57, 123, 130
Aviation, 106

Bande, H.E. Tijjani Muhammad, 56
Bangladesh, 16-19, 22, 24, 32, 43, 47-48, 53, 55, 70-75, 78, 80, 83, 85, 97, 99-101, 105, 109, 134, 162
    Climate Smart Agriculture Investment Plan, 100

    Readymade Garments, 78-79, 82
    Sex Workers Network, 82
Bangladesh, Bhutan and Nepal (BBN), 127
Bangladesh, Bhutan, India and Nepal (BBIN), 127, 130-31
Bangladesh, India and Nepal (BIN), 127
Baru, Rama V., 31
Bay of Bengal Initiative for Multi-Sectoral Technical and Economic Cooperation (BIMST-EC), 127
BBC News, 48, 93, 101, 105, 159
BCIM, 130-31
Bhatia, Rajiv, 133
Bhurgari, Zahid, 50
Bhutan, 16-19, 22, 43, 53, 55, 71, 73, 97, 99-100, 105
Bill & Melinda Gates Foundation, 154, 159
BIMSTEC, 57, 124, 130-33, 135-36, 138-40
Bird Flu, 177
Biruni Institute, 82
Booth, Ken, 4
BRAC, 31
Brazil, 167
Brundtland, G.H., 166
Buzan, Barry, 64
    People, States and Fear, 13, 67

Capitalist Threat, 66
Carbon Emissions, 92
Cedric Habiyaremye, 45
Center, Wilson, 76
Central Pollution Control Board, 104
Centre for Monitoring the Indian Economy (CMIE), 52, 82
Centre for Science and Environment (CSE), *State of India's Environment*, 109

Index

China, 3, 69, 112, 138-39, 142, 149, 157, 167
   physical infrastructure provider, 141
   Belt and Road Initiative (BRI), 139, 142
China-India rivalry, 139
China-Pakistan Economic Corridor, 139
Civil Society, 129-30
Civil Society Organisations (CSOs), 31
Clean Water, Access, 54
Climate Change, 99-100, 105-8, 114-15, 176
Climate Emergency Frontline, 99
Cold War, 5, 12, 64, 66, 94, 126, 148, 165
Commission on Global Governance, 147
Commission on Social Determinants of Health, 168
Communist Threat, 66
Conference of Parties (COP), 107
Confidence-Building Measures (CBMs), 130
Covan, Eleanor Krassen,
   Health Care for Women International, 3, 165
COVID-19 Threatens Global Food Security, 45
Cox's Bazar, 29, 92-93

Dabelko, Geoffrey D., 6
Daily Ittefaq, 50
Dawn, 21
Dhaka Tribune, 47-48, 108-9, 122, 135
Diarrhoea, 55
Dr. Mrinal Sircar, 98
Dr. V.T.H. Gunaratne, 162-63

East Asia, 69
Ebola, 13, 123, 146, 148, 152, 177
Economic Cooperation Organisation (ECO), 128, 131
Economic Growth, 57
Economic Insecurities, 176
Emergency Fund, 134
Environmental Scarcity, 94
Environmental Security, 94
Epstein, Abraham, 5
European Rice Trader, 51
European Union (EU), 123, 130, 138, 140

FAO,
   The State of Food Insecurity in the World 2015, 44
   The State of Food Security and Nutrition in the World 2019, 44
Financial Express, 49, 80
First World War, 150
Fisher, P.B., 6

G-7, 158
Garrett, Laurie, 14
Gates, Bill, 159
George, P.S., 41
Gilpin, 67
Global Alliance for Vaccines and Immunisation (GAVI), 154
Global Burden Project, 98
Global Carbon Emission, 106
Global Developments, 69
Global Economic Recession, 2008, 53
Global Fund (G.F.), 154
Global Health, 147
Global Health Governance (GHG) Institution, 146-49, 157
Global Health Security Index 2019, 165
Global Health Security Risk, 13
Global Leadership, Crisis, 157-59
Globalisation, 130
Gnangnon, Sèna Kimm, 57
Governance, 147
Grandi, Filippo, 100
Growth Triangle (GT) model, 127
Guardian, 39
Gul, Miya, 54
Guterres, António, UN Secretary-General, 29, 157

Hajikhel, Najma, 27
Hardoon, Deborah, 168
Hasina, Sheikh, 100
Hate and Gannon, 15
Health Effects Institute (HEI), 108
Healthcare Privatisation, 20-21
Himal South Asian, 96, 112
Hindustan Times, 47
HIV/AIDS, 28, 123, 152
Hough, Peter, 95
Howard, Julie and Emmy Simmons, 49
Hufbauer, Gary, 57
Human Security, 5-6, 174-75
Husain, Arif, WFP's Chief Economist, 46

IMF, 20, 57, 69, 79
Imperialist Threat, 66
India, 16-19, 22, 32, 43, 47-48, 53, 55, 70-73, 83, 97, 99, 101, 105, 109, 138, 141, 162, 167
  Digital Infrastructure Provider, 141
India Doctrine, 129
Indian Express, 20
Indian Ocean Rim Association (IORA), 128, 131
Indo-Pacific Strategy (IPS), 139
Industry, 106
Information and Communication Technology (ICT), 130
Institute for Health Metrics and Evaluation (IHME), 108
International Energy Agency (IEA), 107
International Health Regulations (IHR) Review Committee, 1, 152, 165
International Labour Organisation, 46
International Sanitary Regulations, 151
Intra-trade, 58
Inzar Gul Safi, 52
IQAir, India, 96
Islam, Shahidul, 135

Japan, 138
Japanese *Asia for the Asians*, 124
Jha, U.C., 113

Karim, Tariq, 131
Kavanagh, Matthew M., 158
Kazakhstan, 56
Khan, Bhutto, 93
Khan, Hayatullah, 63
Khatun, Fahmida, 82

League of Nation's Health Organisation (LNHO), 150
Lockdown, 25, 49, 51, 104, 111
Lodha, Pragya, 26

MacDonald, Adam P., 166
  East Asia Forum, 157
Maciocco & Italian Global Health Watch, 152
Maldives, 16-19, 22, 43, 53, 55, 71, 73, 97, 99-100, 105, 162

Malpass, David, World Bank Group President, 28
Marine Plastic Pollution, 100-1
Mattoo, Aaditya, 156
McGrath, Matt, 105
McInnes, Colin, 12
McKay, Donna, 158
Mehedi Al Amin, 101
Mental Health Issue, 25
Middle East Respiratory Syndrome (MERS), 146
MINDS Foundation, 26
Ministry of Health, India, 52
Modi, Narendra, Prime Minister of India, 133, 135
Mohamed, Amina, 51
Morgenthau, Hans J., 167
Multidimensional Poverty Index (MPI), 72
Myllyvirta, Lauri, 103

National Commission for Women, 29
National Council of Applied Economic Research, Delhi, 52
Natural Disasters, 95
NDTV, 47, 48
Nehru, Former Indian Prime Minister, 124
Nepal, 16-19, 21-22, 43, 53, 55, 70-73, 97, 99-100, 105, 162
Nesadurai, Helen E.S., 68
New Age, 20, 47-48, 104
Ngumbi, Esther, 102
North American Free Trade Agreement (NAFTA), 130
Nuclear Threat Initiative (NTI), 165
Nunes, Joao, 14
Nutrition Access, 54

Office International d'hygiène Publique (OIHP), 149
Overseas Development Aid (ODA), 159
Oxford Poverty and Human Development Initiative (OPHI), 72

Pakistan, 16-19, 22, 32, 43, 53, 55, 70-73, 79, 83, 97, 101, 105, 129, 136, 138
Palit, Amitendu, 77
Pandemic Emergency Purchase Programme (PEPP), 138

Panditaratne, 137
Panu Poutvaara, 46
Papua New Guineans, 28
Peduzzi, Pascal, Director of UNEP/GRID-Geneva, 111
Per Pinstrup-Andersen, 41
Personal Protective Equipment (PPE), 22, 24, 156, 167, 169
Poetzscher, James, 104
Politico-Strategic Cooperation, 128-29
post-COVID-19 world, 178
Power, 106
pre-COVID-19 world, 178
Profits over People, 96, 167

Rabinowicz, Jane & Martin Settle, 46
Rahman, Atiq, 100
Raihan, Selim, 64
Regionalism, 130
Reuters, 40
Risky Business, 94
Rudd, Kevin, 160
Russia, 157
Ruta, Michele, 156

SAARC Comprehensive Framework on Disaster Management, 137
SAARC Preferential Trading Arrangement (SAPTA), 125, 128
Saini, Shweta, 80
Scroll.in, 47, 48
Second World War, 94, 124, 150, 174
Security, 4, 66, 67
Sen, Amartya, 6
Severe Acute Respiratory Syndrome (SARS), 13, 28, 123, 132, 152
Shah, Farzana Altaf, 104
Shukla, Abhay, 21-22, 30
Singh, Sonu, 51
Sino-Indian Doklam Standoff, 139
Sky News, 101
Socio-economic Condition, 25
Soil Degradation, 102
South Asia Co-operative Environment Programme (SACEP), 113
South Asia Economic Focus, 80
South Asia, 2, 4, 7-8
    Basic Drinking Water, 55
    Community Mobility, 105
    Economic Security, 63-87
    Elimination of Diseases in, 164
    Environmental Security, 91-115
    Food Security, 39-59
        People Experienced with Moderate Poor People, 43
        Poverty Headcount Ratio, 43
        Severe Food Insecurity, 44
    GDP Growth, 71
    Health Security, 11-33
        Affected and Deaths, 22
        Births Attended by Skilled Health
        Hospital Beds, 18
        Maternal Mortality Ratio, 19
        Medical Doctors, 17
        Personnel, 19
        Security Studies, 32
    Malaria Incidence, 162
    Sanitation Services, 55
South Asian Alliance for Poverty Eradication (SAAPE), 72
South Asia Inequality Report, 2019, 72
South Asian Association for Regional Cooperation (SAARC), 57-58, 113, 124-27, 130-34, 136-42
South Asian Free Trade Agreement (SAFTA), 125-26, 128, 131
South Asian Growth Quadrangle (SAGQ), 127
South Asian Network on Economic Modelling (SANEM), 80
South Asian Regional Cooperation (SARC), 125
South Asian Sub-regional Economic Cooperation (SASEC), 127, 130-31
Southeast Asia, 69
Soviet Threat, 66
Sri Lanka, 16-19, 22, 43, 53, 55, 70-71, 73, 97, 99-101, 105, 162
Stopford and Strange, 67
Surface Transport, 106
Survival Plus, 4, 67

Tadjbakhsh and Chenoy, 6
The Business Standard, 47-48, 80
The Daily Star, 29, 48, 52, 71-72, 100, 134
The Economic Times, 72, 77, 80-81

The Financial Express, 56
The Hindu, 27, 81, 104
The Indian Express, 47, 97-98, 109
The Japan Times, 63, 93
The New Nation, 48
Thomas Homer-Dixon, 94
Tiensin, *Project Syndicate*, 56
Times of India, 93
Timmer, C. Peter, 41
Toosi, Nahal, 156
Torero, Maximo, 56
Torero, Maximo, Assistant Director-General FAO, 39
Trade Competition, 67
Trump, Donald, U.S. President, 158

Ullman, Richard H., 5
Umar, Asad, 82
UN Food and Agriculture Organisation, 42
UNB News, 47, 104
UNECE, 97
UNICEF, 27, 98, 151
United Nations Development Programme (UNDP), 4-5, 72
   The Human Development Report, 1994, 68
United Nations Development Programme Report, *New Dimensions of Human Security*, 12
United Nations Environment Programme (UNEP), 109

United Nations General Assembly, 45
United Nations World Food Programme, 45
United Nations, 42
USA, 138-39, 149, 157
   Centers for Disease Control and Prevention, 160

Vitamin C, 52

Walt, Stephen M., 4
Washington Post, 158
Wiggings and Slater, 41
World Bank, 20, 27, 44-45, 57, 76, 81, 136, 152-53
World Economic Forum (WEF), 134
World Economic League Table, 70
World Food Conference, 1974, 41
World Food Programme, 49
World Health Organisation (WHO), 1, 3, 12, 18, 29, 96, 110, 146, 149-52, 155, 158-61, 169, 177
Worldometers, 42
Wuhan, 3, 26, 138
Wuhan Virus, 158

Yuk-ping and Thomas, 13

Zaidi, Shehla, 21
Zhao Lijian, 158
Zika, 146, 177